Improving Access to HIV Care

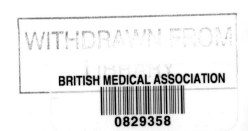

Improving Access to HIV Care

Lessons from Five U.S. Sites

Kriti M. Jain, David R. Holtgrave, Cathy Maulsby, J. Janet Kim,
Rose Zulliger, Meredith Massey, and Vignetta Charles

Johns Hopkins University Press   *Baltimore*

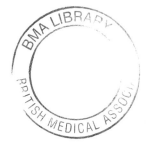

Johns Hopkins University Press
2715 North Charles Street
Baltimore, Maryland 21218-4363
www.press.jhu.edu

Library of Congress Cataloging-in-Publication Data

Jain, Kriti M., 1985– , author.
  Improving access to HIV care : lessons from five U.S. sites /
Kriti M. Jain, David R. Holtgrave, Cathy Maulsby, J. Janet Kim,
Rose Zulliger, Meredith Massey, and Vignetta Charles.
     p. ; cm.
  Includes bibliographical references and index.
  ISBN 978-1-4214-1886-5 (pbk. : alk. paper) — ISBN 978-1-4214-1887-2
(electronic) — ISBN 1-4214-1886-X (pbk. : alk. paper) — ISBN 1-4214-
1887-8 (electronic)
  I. Title.
  [DNLM: 1. HIV Infections—prevention & control—United States—
Case Reports. 2. HIV Infections—therapy—United States—Case
Reports. 3. HIV Long-Term Survivors—United States—Case Reports.
4. Health Services Accessibility—United States—Case Reports. 5. Patient
Acceptance of Health Care—United States—Case Reports. 6. Program
Evaluation—methods—United States—Case Reports. WC 503.2]
  RA643.8
  614.5′99392—dc23   2015012920

A catalog record for this book is available from the British Library.

*Special discounts are available for bulk purchases of this book. For
more information, please contact Special Sales at 410-516-6936 or
specialsales@press.jhu.edu.*

Johns Hopkins University Press uses environmentally friendly book
materials, including recycled text paper that is composed of at least
30 percent post-consumer waste, whenever possible.

To the Positive Charge Intervention Team
for their important public health contributions

Contents

Acknowledgments

The authors would like to express their sincere gratitude to the Positive Charge intervention staff for their dedication and invaluable contributions to this work. We appreciate their graciously sharing their experiences with us through interviews and surveys, as well as reviewing drafts of this book. We would also like to thank the individuals who participated in the PC intervention.

This evaluation project was supported by a grant from AIDS United to Johns Hopkins Bloomberg School of Public Health. The overall Positive Charge Project was supported by a grant from Bristol-Myers Squibb (BMS) to AIDS United. Johns Hopkins Bloomberg School of Public Health had a relationship only with AIDS United (not BMS).

We would also like to acknowledge those who took time to review the manuscript. The findings and conclusions in this volume are those of the authors and do not necessarily represent the views of AIDS United, Johns Hopkins Bloomberg School of Public Health, or the grantees of the Positive Charge initiative.

Improving Access to HIV Care

Introduction

There are approximately 1.2 million people living with HIV (PLWH) in the United States (Centers for Disease Control and Prevention 2012a). Roughly 50,000 individuals are newly diagnosed with HIV annually, and some populations, including younger individuals (20–24 years of age), Black/African Americans, males, and residents of the U.S. South, are disproportionately affected (Centers for Disease Control and Prevention 2012a). The annual rate of death due to HIV infection decreased rapidly from 1994 to 1997 and has continued to decrease steadily (CASCADE Collaboration 2003; Bhaskaran et al. 2008). Currently, this decrease is largely due to the availability of HAART—highly active antiretroviral therapy (Detels et al. 1998; Palella et al. 1998). It stands in stark contrast to the first decades of the HIV epidemic (Torian et al. 2011) as well as the present-day context in many developing countries (World Health Organization 2014). In Europe and North America, the average life expectancies for PLWH continue to increase toward the life expectancy of the general population (Antiretroviral Therapy Cohort Collaboration 2008).

Despite these gains, of the more than one million individuals living with HIV in the United States, more than 50% are not accessing regular care, and this is associated with increased morbidity and mortality (Perkins et al. 2008; Olatosi et al. 2009; Centers for Disease Control and Prevention 2011a, 2013; E. M. Gardner et al. 2011). The United States has set specific goals to stem the epidemic, which are described in the 2010 National HIV/AIDS Strategy. The goals include that, by 2015, 85% of newly diagnosed individuals should be linked to care within three months and 80% of Ryan White HIV/AIDS Program clients should be retained in care. The document also sets goals for decreases in new infections and a greater proportion of PLWH with undetectable viral loads among key populations (ONAP 2010).

Linking PLWH to care and retaining them in care is vital for addressing HIV in the United States (Mugavero et al. 2013). Linkage to and retention in care are associated with decreased viral loads, shorter time between HIV diagnosis and viral suppression, and reduction in HIV transmission to HIV-negative partners (Moore and Bartlett 2011; Althoff et al. 2012; Hall, Gray, et al. 2013). Individuals with suppressed viral loads have a low probability of transmitting HIV and may decrease HIV-risk behaviors (Metsch et al. 2008; Cohen et al. 2011). Furthermore, as drug resistance is increasingly recognized as an obstacle to the prevention benefits of HIV treatment (Gupta et al. 2012; Myerset al. 2012; Cambiano et al. 2014), understanding how to reengage PLWH into HIV care carries increased public health significance.

Barriers to Linkage and Retention

A variety of individual-level factors are associated with delaying or not linking to care. These include substance use, lack of education and information about HIV, and Black/African American ethnicity (Ulett et al. 2009). Psychological factors such as stigma, distress, and fear have also been shown to delay or hinder linkage to care (Kempf et al. 2010; Sprague and Simon 2014). Factors associated with lack of retention in care include Black/African American ethnicity, unstable housing, each additional year of care enrollment, lack of transportation, and baseline CD4 count of greater than 200 cells/μL (Ulett et al. 2009; Kempf et al. 2010; Rebeiro et al. 2013; Haley et al. 2014).

Several structural factors are also associated with not accessing care. These factors include incarceration, lack of transportation, and not meeting basic subsistence needs, such as food and housing (Sprague and Simon 2014). Provider-related factors are also an important component of client engagement. One qualitative study examining this key relationship found that clients prefer providers who are engaging, are validating, see clients as partners in care, and lack paternalistic attitudes (Mallinson et al. 2007).

Factors Associated with Linkage to and Retention in Care

Successfully linking to care is positively associated with several individual-level factors, including a recent HIV diagnosis; reductions in substance use, particularly of cocaine; providing financial support for children within the past six months; older age; disclosure of HIV status; and use of antiretroviral drugs (Wohl, Galvan, et al. 2011; Rebeiro et al. 2013; Haley et al. 2014). Meeting the immediate, basic needs of PLWH also boosted retention in care. Specifically, provision of the following can boost both linkage to and retention in care: nutritional support; health insurance; transportation to appointments; treatment of outstanding mental health conditions; substance use treatment; and access to stable, affordable housing (Andersen et al. 2007; Sprague and Simon 2014). Several studies found that direct, hands-on support for PLWH also boosted retention, whether through psychosocial case management or through dedicated linkage-to-care workers actively linking to care those PLWH who are currently out of care (Conviser and Pounds 2002; Andersen et al. 2007; Wohl, Garland, et al. 2011; Sprague and Simon 2014). Evidence suggests that a positive clinic setting is vital for linkage—specifically, personal relationships with caring and understanding providers; flexible, efficient care; and collocated medical care and social services (Kempf et al. 2010; Sprague and Simon 2014).

Results from Past Linkage and Retention Programs

There are two main studies examining interventions to boost linkage to and engagement in care: the Antiretroviral Treatment and Access to Services (ARTAS) study and the Special Projects of National Significance (SPNS) study, the latter sponsored by the Health Resources and Services Administration (HRSA). ARTAS had a case management (intervention) arm and a control arm. Both arms included HIV education and information about local resources. After one year, 64% of PLWH in the intervention arm were retained in care versus 49% of PLWH in the control group. Factors associated with being linked to care in this study closely mirror those found in other, nonrandomized studies and include an age of 25 years or older, Hispanic ethnicity, being stably housed, no recent use of non-injection drugs, attendance at two or more sessions with the case manager, and recruitment at a site with collocated HIV care (L. I. Gardner et al. 2005; Craw et al. 2008).

The Health Resources and Services Administration's SPNS study on access to care was a ten-site intervention focusing on PLWH in urban areas who are more often left out of care compared with the general population of PLWH (Hall et al. 2012). PLWH were supported in accessing linkage to and retention in care through a variety of context-specific approaches to reduce structural, financial, and personal or cultural barriers to care (Rajabiun et al. 2007). The reduction of substance use was associated with increased retention, and newly diagnosed individuals most often achieved undetectable viral loads. Unlike the findings of previous studies, mental health improvement and decreases in stigma were not associated with improved retention in care, and the presence of stigma remained a barrier to care (Bradford 2007).

Collaboration across Organizations Serving PLWH

Interagency collaboration has been defined as "mutually beneficial and well-defined relationships entered into by two or more organizations to achieve a common goal" (Mattessich and Monsey 1992). Theory suggests that the over-arching aim of interagency collaborations is improved efficiency and performance through the exchange of resources, knowledge, and social capital (Parmigiani and Rivera-Santos 2011). An important attribute of interagency relationships is that they typically involve diverse partners (e.g., community-based organizations, government agencies, and for-profit corporations) with a primary focus on social rather than business issues (Parmigiani and Rivera-Santos 2011). Benefits of collaboration include decreases in duplication of efforts, increases in power and legitimacy, rationalization of resources, and provision of superior services (Lippitt and Van Til 1981; Jones et al. 2004; Parmigiani and Rivera-Santos 2011).

Interagency collaboration can be important for the effective delivery of health services (Dryfoos 1994), particularly in an era when there is increased recognition of the relationship between health outcomes and the "upstream" social factors that have historically been addressed by social support agencies, such as homelessness, joblessness, and substance use. Research on interagency collaboration among HIV service providers has sought to better understand systems of HIV care. A study of thirty agencies in Baltimore suggests that Baltimore's HIV service delivery agencies are relatively well connected and characterizes most of the interagency collaboration as ad hoc rather than structured (Kwait et al. 2001). A study in Indiana that examined mental health services for PLWH found that information sharing was the most frequent type of collaboration (Wright and Shuff 1995). Another study found that during a project requiring collaboration, the types of collaboration that most increased were network referrals, followed by shared resources and information. Network connectedness increased during this project (Provan et al. 2003). In contrast, a study in North Carolina of two HIV-prevention networks found that HIV-prevention agencies were working in isolation, with little interagency collaboration (Thomas et al. 2007). Despite evidence supporting the role of collaboration in solving complex, long-term health issues such as managing HIV, there have been few studies on how to nurture strong, multifaceted collaborations within such networks.

AIDS United's Positive Charge Program

At the time AIDS United's Positive Charge (PC) program launched, many linkage-to-care programs focused on newly diagnosed individuals, and there were few programs for PLWH who had never engaged in care (L. I. Gardner et al. 2005; Naar-King et al. 2007; Craw 2008; Coleman et al. 2009; Hightow-Weidman, Jones, et al. 2011; Hightow-Weidman, Smith, et al. 2011; Wohl et al. 2011). In response, PC focused on PLWH who had never engaged in care, were previously in care, were out of care, or faced significant barriers to care (e.g., substance use, mental health issues, or homelessness). The program focused on underserved populations and aimed to identify the systemic and/or personal barriers to care experienced by PLWH. It also sought to enhance support systems and provide appropriate interventions to alleviate those barriers. PC addressed three goals outlined in the National HIV/AIDS Strategy (NHAS): to reduce the number of people who become infected with HIV, to increase access to HIV care and improve health outcomes for PLWH, and to reduce HIV-related health disparities (ONAP 2010). PC's work particularly addresses the second goal.

PC allowed program models to vary with community needs and available resources. Hence, the structure, model, and strategies differed by site. All sites were required to design their programs based on available evidence. The most common approaches were peer or patient navigation, community health workers, care coordination, and motivational interviewing. Also, to promote sustained improvements in care for PLWH, PC sought to focus on systemic change in addition to addressing individual needs. To do so, PC sites developed collaborative organizational networks to reduce barriers to care and improve the ways in which health and social service systems operate in their community. Throughout this process, Johns Hopkins University collaborated with AIDS United and PC sites to develop and conduct a multifaceted evaluation, which included the case studies featured in this volume.

The purpose of this volume is to examine the process of implementing PC for each of the case study sites and to explore changes in the local network of organizations serving PLWH. Within the implementation process, we seek to answer the following questions: (1) How have subgrantees implemented the following program models/strategies: peer navigation, community health workers, care coordination, and motivational interviewing? (2) What have been the biggest barriers to implementing these models/strategies? (3) What methods have been employed to overcome these barriers successfully? (4) What has facilitated implementation of the models/strategies? (5) What has fostered these facilitating factors? To better understand change at the network level we, first, describe the PC linkage-to-care network at each PC location and, second, assess changes in subcontractor network density and node degree (displayed in sociograms). Finally, we discuss similarities and differences in experiences across the PC sites.

Methods

Setting and Design

AIDS United's Positive Charge (PC) program took place at five locations around the United States. Each location had a lead organization and collaborated with local partners to implement PC. Local partners included medical providers, AIDS service organizations, and social service organizations. All five lead agencies had received a grant from AIDS United to support linkage programs.

The five grantees and their partners sought to link people living with HIV (PLWH) who were out of care to regular medical care. Their programs were tailored to address the needs of out-of-care individuals locally. Each site was in an area severely affected by the HIV epidemic. Lead agencies were selected for grant funding on the basis of their capacity and strong track record in addressing the needs of PLWH in their area. Johns Hopkins University (JHU) supported cross-site evaluation activities, which included the case studies and network analyses presented in this volume.

This volume examines each PC grantee and its network at a single point in time and, as a result, cannot represent the project as a whole or the project at completion. The PC networks evolved as the projects progressed. The five sites were

- *Multiple cities in Louisiana:* In Louisiana, PC was led by the Louisiana Public Health Institute (LPHI) and included 10 partners. The program was implemented in three cities: New Orleans, Baton Rouge, and Lake Charles. Newly diagnosed and out-of-care individuals were the focus for the general population of PLWH. LPHI's PC program also worked extensively with incarcerated or formerly incarcerated individuals.

- *Chicago, IL:* Chicago's PC work was led by the AIDS Foundation of Chicago, which partnered with three other organizations. Their focus was originally on men who have sex with men (MSM) of color but later expanded to include all MSM who were out of care.
- *New York City, NY:* New York City's PC program was led by the New York City AIDS Fund of the New York Community Trust and had nine implementation partners. One of the partners, Amida Care, is a Medicaid Special Needs Plan, and participants were primarily out-of-care individuals enrolled in Amida Care.
- *San Francisco / Bay Area, CA:* The PC site located in San Francisco was led by the Health Equity Institute. It had eight partners. The Bay Area Network for Positive Health focused on multiple high-need populations: men who are or were incarcerated, day laborers, women, injection drug users, and transgender individuals.
- *Multiple regions in North Carolina:* The PC project in North Carolina was led by the Center for Health Policy and Inequalities Research at Duke University, with four other organizations in three regions: rural northeastern region, suburban coastal region, and urban Charlotte. The project sought to engage PLWH who were not already in routine HIV care. (Table 1 gives further details of the five PC sites.)

Each case study includes (1) a basic description of its PC project and its context; (2) a diagram of the network of organizations involved; (3) sociograms of agency collaboration before and during PC; and (4) insights about the process of program implementation, drawing on qualitative data. A sociogram is a chart that plots relationships between entities, in this case organizations. Each node represents an organization. A line between nodes indicates that organizations worked together to link PLWH to care. Mixed-methods case study is an appropriate research method to evaluate PC implementation because the PC project is "a contemporary phenomenon in depth and within its real life context, especially when the boundaries between phenomenon and context are not clearly evident," where "the investigator has little or no control" (Yin 2009).

The specific study design is an embedded, multiple-case study. Each of the five PC programs constitutes a "case," and within each of the five programs, each organization (lead and partners) is an embedded unit of analysis within

Table 1 Positive Charge site descriptions and timelines

Lead organization	Program name	Program population and linkage strategy	Implementation start date
Louisiana Public Health Institute (LPHI)	Louisiana Positive Charge Initiative	Newly diagnosed people living with HIV (PLWH); individuals out of care for 1 year or longer; PLWH at risk of falling out of care; LPHI focused on men, minorities, persons 25–44 years of age, residents of selected cities	Aug 2010
AIDS Foundation of Chicago	Project IN-CARE	Out-of-care PLWH and MSM (men who have sex with men) of color; later expanded to all MSM	Aug 2010
New York City AIDS Fund of the New York Community Trust	ACCESS NY	PLWH who are low-income residents of the Bronx, Brooklyn, and Manhattan	Aug 2011
Health Equity Institute for Research, Policy, and Practice (San Francisco State University)	Bay Area Network for Positive Health (BANPH)	Out-of-care (or at risk of falling out of care) PLWH living in poverty, recently incarcerated, who are substance users, transgender, or people of color	Aug 2011
Center for Health Policy and Inequalities Research at Duke University	North Carolina Positive Charge Initiative	Out-of-care (or at risk of falling out of care) PLWH who are aware of their status	July 2010

a larger program (Yin 2009). To the extent possible, we sought to use emic terminology. For example, each site used its own terminology to refer to staff who worked directly with clients to provide nonclinical services and who may themselves have been PLWH (e.g., "peer navigators," who were often PLWH, or "access coordinators"). In presenting each of the five case studies, we use the emic term used by the interviewees. In the discussions and conclusions of this volume, however, we use the term "peer" for clarity.

This book aims to provide a snapshot of each PC grantee and its network at one point in time. It is not representative of the project as a whole or of the project at its completion. Rather, networks, like interventions, are dynamic and evolve over time. The case studies were part of a three-pronged evaluation that included client outcomes and economic analyses (Kim et al. 2014; Maulsby et al. 2015). No individual client data were handled by JHU, and the university's institutional review board (IRB) did not consider this study to be human subjects research. Individual sites received IRB approval from their relevant local institutions. There were no incentives for participating in any part of the case studies.

Data Collection

Data collection methods for the case studies included document reviews, qualitative interviews, online surveys, and participatory documentation.

Document Reviews

The PC evaluation team, based at Johns Hopkins Bloomberg School of Public Health, Department of Health, Behavior and Society, reviewed available documentation related to each PC grantee site, including PC site proposals, reports by key health agencies on HIV in the local area, epidemiological data, agency websites, and reports by implementing agencies.

Qualitative Data Collection

Qualitative data were collected by JHU evaluation staff using in-depth, semi-structured interviews. Interviewees were selected through purposive sampling. Where possible, two people were interviewed at each lead and each partner organization. To capture a variety of perspectives and activities, one of the individuals worked at the administrative level (e.g., an AIDS service organization director) and the other directly provided services to clients (e.g., a peer health navigator). Evaluators at JHU worked closely with grantees to identify and set up appointments with appropriate individuals to interview.

During each interview, each respondent was asked about the process of linking clients to and retaining them in care, changes within the organization as a result of the linkage and retention project, challenges to implementation, facilitating factors, changes in interorganizational collaboration, and the impact of policy on linkage and retention work. The full semistructured interview guide is available as appendix A. Each interview lasted between 45 and

90 minutes and was conducted by a single interviewer, either in person or on the phone. The interviewer was a JHU-based evaluator. The number of interviews was determined by the number of partners involved in the program and by the availability of interviewees (table 2). Across all five grantee sites, forty interviews were conducted. All interviews were audio-recorded and transcribed.

Online Survey Data Collection

To explore interorganizational connectivity, network analysis data were collected through an online survey. To the extent possible, the same individuals who participated in the in-depth interviews also took the online survey (table 2). The survey questions asked which organizations were working together at the time of the survey, which had been collaborating organizations six months before project implementation, and in what capacities organizations were collaborating. Respondents with supervisory responsibilities ("administrative") had an additional survey section containing questions on organizational resources, such as funding and the number of employees.

The questions were adapted from two sources: Messeri and Kiperman 1994 and Kwait et al. 2001. Reliability and validity testing was not conducted. However, these questions have strong face validity and were reviewed by various experts in the field. In addition, asking respondents about a "checklist" of possible collaborating organizations they worked with is a widely used method for collecting network data (Messeri and Kiperman 1994; Kwait et al. 2001). These questions are included as appendix B.

Participatory Diagramming

In addition to the in-depth interviews and online surveys, the agencies and JHU-based evaluators created network graphics, using a two-step process. Initially, each lead agency drafted its network graphic during a participatory exercise held at an all-grantee meeting in 2010. This network graphic was then updated in October 2011, before the in-depth interviews, with multiple rounds of review between JHU-based evaluators and PC grantees.

Analysis
Qualitative Data

The analysis employed conventional content analysis (Hsieh and Shannon 2005). In-depth interviews were read completely and analyzed using inductive coding to examine the categories within the broader themes of linkage to

Table 2 Data collected by Positive Charge sites

PC site	Number of interviews	Organizations interviewed	Interview dates	Number of surveys	Organizations surveyed	Survey dates
Multiple cities, Louisiana	9* Admin: 6 Service: 5	Capitol Area Reentry Program HIV Outpatient Program (HOP) Clinic NO/AIDS Task Force Louisiana Office of Public Health Moss Regional Hospital N'R Peace Orleans Parish Prison Southwest Louisiana AIDS Council	June–July 2011	20 Admin: 12 Service: 8	Capitol Area Reentry Program Earl K. Long Medical Center HOP clinic NO/AIDS Task Force Louisiana Office of Public Health Louisiana Public Health Institute Moss Regional Hospital N'R Peace Orleans Parish Prison Southwest Louisiana AIDS Council	May–Dec 2011
Chicago	7 Admin: 4 Service: 3	AIDS Foundation of Chicago CORE Center Howard Brown Health Center Test Positive Aware Network	Feb 2012	5 Admin: 4 Service: 1	AIDS Foundation of Chicago CORE Center Howard Brown Health Center Test Positive Aware Network	June 2012–Mar 2013

Location	N	Breakdown	Organizations	Date	N	Breakdown	Organizations	Date
New York City	6	Admin: 4 Service: 2	Amida Care Callen-Lorde Community Health Center HELP PSI Primary Care Development Corporation	Oct 2012	6	Admin: 4 Service: 2	Amida Care Callen-Lorde Community Health Center HELP PSI Primary Care Development Corporation	Dec 2012–June 2013
San Francisco/Bay Area	11	Admin: 5 Service: 6	Alameda County Department of Public Health Centerforce Forensic AIDS Project Health Equity Institute San Francisco AIDS Foundation Street Level Health Project Women Organized to Respond to Life Threatening Diseases (WORLD)	Sep 2011	12	Admin: 9 Service: 3	Alameda County Department of Public Health Centerforce Forensic AIDS Project Health Equity Institute Mission Neighborhood Health Center Street Level Health Project WORLD	Nov–Dec 2011
Multiple regions, North Carolina	8	Admin: 4 Service: 4	AIDS Care and Education Services Hertford County Public Health Authority Mecklenburg County Health Department Regional AIDS Interfaith Network	Sep 2011	10	Admin: 4 Service: 6	AIDS Care and Education Services Hertford County Public Health Authority Mecklenburg County Health Department	Sep 2011–Jun 2012

*Two interviews were conducted with two respondents simultaneously.

and retention in care programs. Initially, open coding was conducted. Categories and category names arising from the data formed the basis of initial codes, which were then sorted into clusters. Inductive coding allowed exploration of new ideas and themes emerging from the data that were not originally anticipated. ATLAS.ti software was used to assign and organize codes (ATLAS.ti 2013). Three different researchers analyzed the data from different sites, but all used the same coding guide to ensure consistency across individual site data analysis. The coding guide was developed collaboratively by two researchers.

To enhance trustworthiness of findings, coding and findings were reviewed across interviewers and by other evaluation team members (Lincoln and Guba 1985). All team members had significant prior experience in developing and coding qualitative content. In describing the findings, terminology specific to each site was used (e.g., "access coordinator" or "peer health navigator"). Quotes were anonymized at two levels (speaker and organization) to preserve confidentiality. An internal audit was conducted through iterative reviews of findings with both lead and partner organizations (Manning 1997). Each organization reviewed its site's individual section of the case studies both in the early stages, soon after interviews were conducted, and at the final stages of writing.

Online Surveys

Network analysis relied on survey data, which were converted to matrices for analysis. The matrices included the lead and partner organizations as headers in each row and column, and a 1 or 0 indicated whether or not collaboration was reported between the organizations named in that row and column: 1 signified reported collaboration, and 0 meant that no collaboration was reported. For sites with complete survey data, nonreciprocal ties could be included in the analysis (sociogram, density, and network centralization). For sites with incomplete data, ties were assumed to be bidirectional. That is, if one organization reported collaboration with another, it was assumed to be reciprocal. Incomplete surveys were discarded, and if one individual had completed multiple surveys, only the most recent was used. These matrices were then loaded into UCINET to calculate network centralization, average node degree, and density before and during the PC project. The sociograms, which were used to visualize the network before and during PC, were created using UCINET's companion software, NetDraw (Borgatti et al. 2002).

Executive Summaries
of Case Study Findings

Multiple Cities, Louisiana

The Louisiana Positive Charge (PC) network identified out-of-care people living with HIV (PLWH) and linked them to and retained them in HIV primary care. The network comprised ten organizations: three Louisiana State University clinics, a public health institute, a health department, a county jail, and four community-based organizations. The project took place in three distinct geographic areas of Louisiana: New Orleans, Baton Rouge, and Lake Charles.

Changes to the Louisiana Positive Charge Network

Before implementation of the Louisiana PC, there were few connections among partner organizations. The network had a density of 0.30, or 27 of 90 possible connections between organizations were reported. During PC, the network became highly interconnected, despite the project's three distinct geographic locations. The density of the network increased to 0.69. In other words, 62 of 90 possible connections between organizations existed.

Project Implementation

Each organization indicated that it had undergone internal structural changes as a result of PC. By the end of the project, eight of the ten organizations had staff housed in a partner organization or housed staff from a partner organization. These relationships facilitated improvements in systems for referrals, identification, intake, and appointments.

Linkage to care required significant collaboration among agencies. Organizations reported that the most successful identification systems relied heavily on information sharing among organizations. In many cases, these systems were developed jointly by two or more partner organizations and were improved over time through ongoing monitoring, assessment, and adjustment.

Linkage was more successful when supported by strong relationships across organizations. Respondents described improvements such as being able to link clients to a specific individual within an organization rather than referring to the organization and being more specialized in the linkages they made (e.g., based on a clients' insurance needs or on location of the clinic).

Organizations reported that creating close intra- and interorganizational relationships took significant effort. Health navigators indicated that there was a period of adjustment before they felt fully integrated. Taking the time to understand partner organizations' needs facilitated successful program planning. This communication was particularly critical at the management level. Similarly, open communication between health care staff and peer navigators / post-release case managers allowed more successful collaboration.

Another important finding was the necessity of addressing clients' unmet needs. According to health navigators, successful linkage required first working with clients to address the barriers that kept them from care. The most frequently cited barrier was transportation, followed by mental health issues, substance use, joblessness, and poverty. When staff were asked what they needed to do their jobs better, they mentioned transportation and support services for PLWH in the areas mentioned as barriers above, as well as housing. Sites also noted staffing needs in the areas of data collection and retention in care.

Overarching Conclusions

Through strong interorganizational collaboration in the Louisiana PC, clients' needs were better addressed because the services provided could be tailored to their individual situations. Several factors supported this change, including management-level staff's improved understanding of partner organizations' needs and open communication to clarify the roles of frontline staff across organizations. Through PC, partner organizations had developed tight collaborations, including housing staff at each other's organizations.

Significant barriers to care did remain, however. Health navigators often described insufficient resources to help clients address barriers to HIV care, such as substance use and lack of mental health care. Sites also reported needing greater resources for transportation. Future linkage-to-care programs could benefit from including an even larger support service component.

Chicago

Project Identify, Navigate, Connect, Access, Retain, and Evaluate (IN-CARE) was a consortium comprising one central agency and three implementation partners. This intervention model aimed to facilitate access to and retention in care of men who have sex with men (MSM) living with HIV in Chicago, using a peer-led approach.

Changes to the Chicago Positive Charge Network

During PC implementation, this already tight network stayed connected. Each network partner reported working with all of the others, resulting in the highest possible density—a density of 1, before and during PC.

Project Implementation

Despite citing a few barriers and challenges to program implementation, study respondents valued Project IN-CARE. They mentioned using project data, for the first time, to develop programs. Organizations also mentioned that they benefited from the collaboration and buy-in from network partners that were cultivated at the outset of planning of the PC project.

One respondent described the innovative nature of the project: "IN-CARE was really sort of the first peer program at four distinct agencies with a very distinct intervention that demonstrated that there could be potentially an impact by having peers working with individuals" (Org. A). Respondents consistently described the value of the peer-based approach. They thought that the work of peers and the emphasis on linkage and retention positively influenced the work they were doing and were now integral components of their care model. By staying in contact with clients from the time they were diagnosed until stabilization in care, Project IN-CARE peers were able to improve the quality of care provided for clients and decrease the case burden for case managers. There was initial tension between these care providers, but this seemed to be resolved through clarification of the different cadres' tasks.

Respondents highlighted the value of Project IN-CARE within their own services, but felt that they continued to work independently in silos. They expressed frustration about the lack of communication from project management and thought they would benefit from increased networking and collaboration across organizations. They also emphasized a need to streamline data entry mechanisms and to provide project materials in Spanish.

Overarching Conclusions

Overall, the organizations in the Chicago PC project reported that they were able to address the needs of MSM living with HIV in Chicago and enhance linkage to and retention in care.

New York City

ACCESS NY was a consortium of three key collaborators (New York City AIDS Fund of the New York Community Trust, Amida Care, and Primary Care Development Corporation) and seven primary care provider partners (Housing Works, HELP PSI / Project Samaritan, Callen-Lorde, Village Care of New York, Acacia Network, Harlem United, and St. Mary's Episcopal Center). ACCESS NY had two objectives: (1) to provide primary medical care for Medicaid-eligible PLWH in New York City who were not receiving care and (2) to strengthen the service systems for primary care providers, allowing clients to be retained in care.

Changes to the New York City Positive Charge Network

Implementation of ACCESS NY led to a new focus among the project partners on retaining clients in HIV primary care through the work of peer staff, who did intensive work to find or reengage clients. A department within one agency shifted its focus to retention and care and, with support from additional grants, grew from one to twenty people during the project implementation period. Several new projects were built from this experience. Through the intervention, there was also greater collaboration both within the lead agency and across all of the partner agencies, particularly through structured, cross-site meetings in the Primary Care Development Corporation's Learning Collaborative.

Project Implementation

Engagement in the Learning Collaborative was another main component of this intervention, and it aimed to improve clinical systems to allow better access to and retention in care. During meetings of the collaborative, clinical partners shared their experiences and challenges and worked to modify processes at their clinics to boost access for clients served by ACCESS NY. New techniques for identification and linkage were also explored, such as working with clients who were soon to be discharged from the hospital.

A key challenge in project implementation was that clients were challenging to find, often did not want to seek care, and faced multiple competing barriers. Some of these barriers, such as housing, were particularly challenging to address in the context of New York City. Some of the project implementation procedures were challenging for staff, such as the 30-day limit for linking clients to care. Other challenges for project staff were related to data management tools and timely, complete reporting. The lead agency's data system was not designed to handle such a large volume of data and variables. It was also difficult to train staff in understanding and collecting the data, both for the PC evaluation deliverables and for the Learning Collaborative.

Overarching Conclusions

Despite the challenges in the New York PC project, respondents reported positive reactions from clients. Respondents were enthusiastic and believed in the ACCESS NY program. Following its successful implementation, several of the organizations have continued to build on this work.

San Francisco / Bay Area

The Bay Area Network for Positive Health (BANPH) consisted of nine organizations that collaborated to link out-of-care PLWH to regular medical care as part of a five-site initiative. The network included a diverse set of entities, including two health departments, five community-based social service organizations, a health center, and an academic institution.

All members of BANPH worked with different, underserved populations, including day laborers, women, and formerly incarcerated individuals. BANPH partners used several strategies to identify individuals who were out of care, including referrals, in-reach, and outreach.

Changes to the Bay Area Positive Charge Network

The BANPH organizations became more connected during PC. The network density increased from 0.25 before PC to 0.64 during PC. The BANPH organizations reported that the most common types of collaboration involved attending regularly scheduled joint meetings, exchanging information by phone and email, and discussing services offered by BANPH network partners with their clients.

Project Implementation

At the organizational level, the most widely reported internal structural change resulting from BANPH was hiring staff to conduct outreach and linkage-to-care work. Organizations stressed the importance of addressing participants' needs and priorities as a way to tackle the issues that were keeping clients out of care and to build rapport with clients. Clients had multiple and often interrelated needs, such as for mental health and substance use services, and the most pressing need that emerged was housing.

The quality of relationships between linkage workers and participants was critical to the program's success. In addition, relationships among organizations emerged as an important theme. Strong relationships among organizations facilitated identification of individuals who were out of care, linkage to HIV primary care appointments, linkage to support services, and retention in care. Strong relationships also strengthened channels of communication among organizations, specifically with regard to referrals and follow-up.

BANPH faced some barriers to program implementation. For example, navigating new systems such as prisons was challenging in the beginning. BANPH sought out the most underserved clients, which created challenges because of their burden of need, which included substance use, mental health services, poverty, homelessness, and pervasive stigma.

Overarching Conclusions

Overall, BANPH was a successful program that linked a particularly underserved population, facing many barriers, to ongoing medical care. Organizations used multiple methods, including outreach, to identify potential clients. Fostering relationships between program staff and clients and addressing urgent client needs (e.g., mental health and substance use services) were seen as key to success. Housing, however, posed one of the toughest barriers to care, especially given the relatively expensive housing and rental market in the Bay Area.

Developing relationships among organizations to foster collaboration was particularly important because it facilitated referrals. While network analysis showed an increase in organizational connectedness through PC, organizations indicated a desire to work more closely with their BANPH network partners. This represents a potential area of growth for the BANPH network. Having memoranda of understanding between BANPH network organizations may aid this level of collaboration.

Multiple Regions in North Carolina

The North Carolina Positive Charge network comprised five organizations that worked to boost linkage to and retention in HIV care. The organizations were located in different regions of the state, including the rural northeastern region, suburban coastal region, and urban Charlotte/Mecklenburg County. Of the five organizations, one provided funding and technical assistance, and the other four provided services to individuals living with HIV.

Changes to the North Carolina Positive Charge Network

Before implementation of the PC project, organizations worked only with other groups in their immediate geographic region. Over time, the North Carolina PC network became denser as organizations formed more connections with one another. Before PC, the network density was 0.40; during PC, the network density was 0.80.

Project Implementation

Effective linkage to care required collaboration and flexibility in partnerships. Organizations relied heavily on information sharing among agencies to identify individuals who were never in care or currently out of care. Few organizations successfully identified potential clients without information sharing. In many cases, these relationships were established before the start of the PC program. Successful linkage to care also often relied heavily on informal relationships and on particular individuals who had experience working with the local population of PLWH. Partners that were unable to establish relationships found creative ways to identify their intended population, including through education, outreach, and support groups.

All sites reported positive structural changes as a result of their partnering with the PC project. PC enabled partner organizations to increase the number of staff and to offer more services, which enabled them to more effectively serve PLWH in their communities. The role of peers—who were often individuals living with HIV—in working with clients was seen as instrumental to PC's success.

Findings from this study support the necessity of addressing clients' unmet needs. Sites indicated a dearth of support services for PLWH in the areas of mental health treatment, housing, substance use treatment, and job placement. These persistent needs were seen as barriers to care.

The most frequently cited barrier to care was transportation. Particularly in rural areas, services are spread out, and lack of transportation can keep PLWH from accessing the services available to them. One site used mobile units to meet clients, conduct CD4 and viral load tests, and review the results with clients. For medical appointments, access coordinators were willing to transport clients, but some agencies' internal policies prevented them from doing so. Access coordinators who were allowed to drive clients to appointments found that the long distances in their own cars, without reimbursement, were a significant burden.

Sites also noted a need for more providers. In rural areas, service providers, including primary care and infectious disease specialists, were spread out geographically and difficult to reach. In the urban area, there were not enough providers.

Overarching Conclusions

Following implementation of the North Carolina PC program, partnering organizations collaborated more across regions, as evidenced by the higher network density. The organizations most successful in locating and linking out-of-care individuals to HIV care were those that formed successful partnerships, often based on informal connections between individuals. Organizations' capacity and reach increased because of PC. The work of peer navigators, in particular, was seen as contributing to success.

Linkage-to-care programs should be designed to address barriers to care such as transportation and unmet client needs. Programs should include a significant, integrated support service component, including for basic client needs such as transportation to appointments, mental health care, housing, job placement, and substance use treatment. Lack of available providers remains a structural issue hindering the success of linkage-to-care programs.

Overall Findings

For the five case study sites, experiences with PC and linkage to care had many parallels: all hired additional staff, increased their focus on linkage to care, increased their collaboration across partner agencies, found that unmet client needs were far greater than anticipated and were often psychosocial (e.g., distrust of the medical system), and expended significant time and energy on locating clients because their contact information often changed. Respondents from several sites described geography-specific issues such as lack of transportation, the challenge of navigating systems such as prisons, and lack of adequate social support services. Several sites discussed early struggles with organizational issues such as data management and staff turnover. All sites, however, reported that the role of peers was vital to the success of their programs. Peers' passion and dedication were universally lauded, despite the challenges of clearly differentiating the roles of peer and case manager.

The experiences reported in this book were pioneering as these five sites began their linkage-to-care work at a time when few such programs existed. We believe that these trailblazing experiences are extremely valuable for future groups conducting similar work, and based on their experiences, we compiled the following recommendations:

1. Recognize and plan for a complex constellation of client needs.
2. Nurture and cultivate interorganizational networks despite inevitable challenges.
3. Proactively establish procedures to share information about clients or potential clients.
4. Create strong relationships with medical providers.
5. Involve peers or other health navigators to support clients in linking to care.
6. Maintain ongoing organizational management.

Multiple Cities in the State of Louisiana

Background

In 2011, Louisiana had the third-highest HIV diagnosis rate of all U.S. states, the District of Columbia, and six dependent areas at 30.2 per 100,000 individuals and the fourth-highest AIDS diagnosis rate at 18.4 per 100,000. There were 17,411 people living with HIV and AIDS in Louisiana, 53% of whom had an AIDS diagnosis (Centers for Disease Control and Prevention 2011a). In the same year, the Baton Rouge metropolitan area ranked first among metropolitan statistical areas of residence in the United States and Puerto Rico for estimated AIDS case rates, and New Orleans–Metairie–Kenner ranked fourth. HIV disproportionately affected Black/African Americans in Louisiana, with 74% of the burden of HIV incidence and 76% of new AIDS cases occurring among this population (Louisiana Office of Public Health [LA OPH] 2011).

Louisiana has a comprehensive public hospital system that provides inpatient and outpatient medical services through eight regional Louisiana State University (LSU) hospitals. Managed by the Health Care Services Division, these LSU facilities admit more than 50,000 patients annually and provide nearly 1.2 million outpatient visits. This hospital system provides the care for many persons who are uninsured in Louisiana (LSU 2009). In addition, the Office of Public Health (OPH) provides a variety of free and low-cost health services, including family planning, HIV testing, screening and treatment of sexually transmitted infections (STIs), maternal and child health, special health services for children, nutrition programs, and immunizations (LA OPH 2011). In 2009, Medicaid or Medicare covered approximately one-third of persons living in Louisiana (Department of Health and Hospitals State of Louisiana 2015; U.S. Census Bureau 2015).

Louisiana received about $65 million in HIV and AIDS grant funding in 2009 from the Centers for Disease Control and Prevention, Housing Opportunities for Persons with AIDS, Substance Abuse and Mental Health Services Administration, and Office of Minority Health HIV and AIDS Funding. The state received about $46 million in Ryan White HIV/AIDS Program funding in FY 2010, and more than $21 million of that funding went toward AIDS Drug Assistance Program (ADAP) expenditures (Kaiser Family Foundation 2012). In 2010, ADAP in Louisiana served 3,557 people living with HIV (PLWH). Of the recipients, 62% were Black/African American and 70% were male. Louisiana has syringe exchange programs in two cities (amfAR 2013).

Program Overview

The Louisiana Positive Charge (PC) network was a ten-agency partnership that aimed to improve linkage to and retention in HIV care and to provide supportive services for newly diagnosed and out-of-care PLWH in three cities. The collaboration was led by the Louisiana Public Health Institute and included health centers, community-based organizations (CBOs), and government agencies. To identify potential clients, PC relied on out-of-care client lists at clinics and HIV-specific disease intervention specialists working in STI clinics and public testing sites. The Louisiana Public Health Information Exchange (LaPHIE) also helped to identify potential clients. LaPHIE is a system that allowed effective, rapid, and secure exchange of client health information among LSU public hospitals, community-based health care providers, and OPH (Herwehe et al. 2011).

To link and retain clients, PC used slightly different strategies in each location, and these included a brief, intense, and strengths-based case management model (Antiretroviral Treatment and Access to Services), health educators and health navigators located in hospitals, a post-release case manager focused on former prison inmates, and a community-based peer health navigator.

Positive Charge Partner Organizations

The Positive Charge network in Louisiana consisted of ten partner agencies in New Orleans, Baton Rouge, and Lake Charles. These organizations collaborated to support individuals living with HIV to receive medical care. The network comprised the OPH STI/HIV/AIDS Program, three LSU public hospital clinics, four community-based organizations, a county jail, and a public health institute, all described below as they existed at the time of the case study.

1. *Louisiana Public Health Institute (LPHI):* LPHI is the lead agency for AIDS United's PC initiative. The institute aims to improve population-level

health outcomes by coordinating and managing a variety of public health programs in the areas of health promotion, disease prevention, and health systems development. LPHI's program focuses on a diverse range of health needs, including maternal and child health, teen pregnancy, tobacco use, and wellness.

2. *Office of Public Health STI/HIV/AIDS Program (OPH)*: The Office of Public Health's STI/HIV/AIDS Program (HAP; later renamed the STD and HIV Program, SHP) coordinates statewide and regional programs to prevent HIV transmission, increases access to medical and social services for PLWH, and conducts statewide HIV surveillance. HAP also works with various CBOs to provide a range of HIV prevention programs, including HIV counseling and testing, development of educational materials, and programs for PLWH, as well as outreach and training activities. In addition, HAP provides services such as primary medical care, medication assistance, case management, hospice care, support services (housing, legal assistance, transportation, nutrition), and assistance with insurance payments. Surveillance activities include case ascertainment though reports from clinical providers, laboratories, and other public health providers. PLWH served by OPH are predominantly Black/African American and between the ages of 35 and 55 years.

In addition, OPH maintains the Louisiana Public Health Information Exchange. The system works by including reminders to clinicians within patients' electronic health records, flagging any pending HIV care for that patient.

3. *HIV Outpatient Program (HOP)*: HOP is an established ambulatory care department under the Interim LSU Public Hospital located in New Orleans. Started in 1987, the primary focus of HOP has been the care and treatment of PLWH, support and coordination for partners, disease prevention, research, and health promotion. HOP delivers clinical and educational services and conducts research. The multidisciplinary clinic provides a wide range of services, including primary care, social services, health and adherence education, pharmaceutical consultation, nutrition services, lab services, and medical subspecialty clinics such as psychiatry, pulmonology, ophthalmology, dermatology, dental care, and gynecology. HOP's clients are primarily urban, low-income, Black/African American, and male, and are Medicare or Medicaid insured or uninsured.

4. *Earl King Long Medical Center (EKL)*: EKL is an acute care hospital that serves patients in East Baton Rouge Parish and the seven surrounding parishes. (The center closed on April 14, 2013; its clinics are now managed by

LSU Health Baton Rouge [LSU Health 2015].) EKL provides primary medical care through four clinics in the area and provides outpatient services for women's health, family practice, internal medicine, surgery, orthopedics, oral surgery, HIV care, pediatrics, dermatology, and other subspecialties. The medical center provides inpatient services for obstetrics, internal medicine, emergency medicine, and surgery. EKL served approximately 79,000 patients from 2006 to 2008.

5. *W. O. Moss Medical Center (Moss):* The Dr. Walter O. Moss Regional Medical Center serves patients in Lake Charles. The hospital provides a wide range of services, including diagnostic radiology, nutritional services, emergency medicine, nuclear medicine, nursing services, pathology and lab services, inpatient and outpatient pharmacy, respiratory care, and social services.

6. *Capitol Area Re-entry Program (CARP):* CARP is a minority-owned community-based organization located in Baton Rouge in an area identified by OPH as a priority zip code due to need. CARP's mission is to provide comprehensive services to underserved and disadvantaged populations, including PLWH, ex-offenders, men who have sex with men, transgender populations, high-risk heterosexuals, homeless populations, injection drug users, and incarcerated individuals. The organization provides a range of support services to PLWH, as well as HIV education, HIV prevention, and smoking cessation.

7. *N'R Peace (NRP):* N'R Peace is a nonprofit community-based organization providing health education and HIV- and AIDS-related services throughout New Orleans. The agency works primarily with PLWH of color who are not currently taking medications, using substances, or homeless, and who have limited access to health information and health care. In addition to providing primary medical care, NRP provides health education, community outreach, free HIV testing, free syphilis screening, peer support programs, Medicaid case management, prevention case management, early intervention services, pregnancy prevention education for teens, and Medicaid enrollment appointments.

8. *Southwest Louisiana AIDS Council (SLAC):* SLAC is a nonprofit community-based organization that provides HIV prevention and a variety of other services to PLWH. SLAC's mission is to provide education to the people of Southwest Louisiana about HIV, AIDS, and HIV prevention and to offer assistance to those affected by the disease. SLAC's programs include HIV education, free HIV testing, case management, support groups, and support services such as a food pantry. The client community served by SLAC is rural

individuals of low socioeconomic status and with high rates of illiteracy. About one-third of SLAC's clients are minorities.

9. *NO/AIDS Task Force:* NO/AIDS Task Force is a community-based organization with a mission to reduce the spread of HIV infection, provide social services, advocate for empowerment, safeguard the rights and dignity of HIV-affected individuals, and provide for an enlightened public. NO/AIDS offers more than twenty programs in four locations throughout New Orleans and the Houma/Thibodeaux area. Its HIV medical clinic provides primary care for HIV and AIDS and related chronic conditions.

10. *Orleans Parish Sheriff's Office (Orleans Parish Prison) Medical Department (OPP):* Orleans Parish Sheriff's Office, referred to as OPP or the Orleans Parish Prison, is a county jail that provides for the care, custody, and control of incarcerated individuals in Orleans Parish. The medical department maintains a full-time nursing staff, with services to six clinics, specialty psychiatric and medical units, and the intake and processing center. Primary medical, dental, and psychiatric care are provided on-site, as are HIV and tuberculosis care. Full-spectrum specialty care is provided at the LSU Health Sciences Center (Charity Hospital and its satellites). Here, patients attend outpatient clinics, receive specialty radiological and surgical services, and are occasionally hospitalized. Routine lab and radiology services are available at the jail, and teams of ancillary professionals conduct tuberculosis testing, STI/HIV testing, and health education.

Tables 3 and 4 summarize the characteristics of the PC sites and the services offered to clients.

Louisiana Positive Charge Network
Network Graphic

Figure 1 shows the Louisiana PC network. Organizations are represented by boxes. Gray boxes indicate the role each organization played in the linkage-to-care continuum—identification of PLWH who are out of care, outreach and linkage to care, provision of HIV primary care, and provision of support services. As represented by the long box at the top of the figure, LPHI is the lead agency for PC in Louisiana; it oversaw and coordinated PC linkage-to-care activities. The Louisiana PC project employed three linkage-to-care strategies: OPH disease intervention specialist (DIS) officers, health navigators, and a pre/post-release case manager. Reading from the top left of the

Table 3 Positive Charge network partners, Louisiana

Organization	Legal fiscal designation	Type of health service agency	Annual HIV operation budget	Number of PLWH served, 2010	Number of paid employees, 2010	Number of volunteers, 2010
LPHI	Private nonprofit	Statewide public health institute	$26,000,000 (overall; not only HIV)	1,200*	85	8
OPH	Public	Health department	$46,000,000	4,000	75	10
HOP	Public	Hospital-based clinic	$7,220,727	2,400	56	0
EKL	Public	Hospital-based clinic	$1,600,000	1,300–1,556	26	0
Moss	Public	Hospital-based clinic	$1,700,000	470	300	15
CARP	Private	Community-based organization	$91,000	100	4	3
NRP	Private nonprofit	Community-based organization	$305,000	390	17	26
SLAC	Private nonprofit	AIDS service organization	$1,236,100	330	24	30–40
NO/AIDS Task Force	Private nonprofit	Community-based organization	$10,000,000	2,000	130	300
OPP	Public	County jail	$5,000,000 (for all medical, not only HIV)	906	55 (in medical)	2

Note: All organization names are given in full in the text.
*Served by grantees; LPHI did not provide services to clients.

Table 4 Services offered to PLWH by PC partner organizations, Louisiana

Organization	STI/HIV counseling and testing	HIV primary care	HIV case management	HIV outreach and linkage to care	HIV peer support	Other health services	Counseling services	HIV education and prevention services	Assistance with entitlement services	Support services*
OPH	×	×	×	×	×	×		×	×	H, T, N
HOP	×	×		×		×	×	×	×	T, N, ID, MH
EKL	×	×	×		×	×	×	×	×	T, S
Moss	×	×	×	×	×	×	×	×	×	H, S
CARP				×	×			×	×	T, ID
NRP	×	×		×		×	×	×	×	
SLAC	×		×	×	×	×	×	×	×	H, T, N, S, C
NO/AIDS Task Force	×	×	×	×	×	×	×	×	×	H, T, N, S
OPP	×	×		×		×		×	×	H, S

Note: LPHI is a funder, not a service provider, so is not included in this table. All organization names are given in full in the text.

*C = child care; H = housing; ID = ID cards; MH = mental health services; N = nutritional support or food; S = substance use treatment; T = transportation.

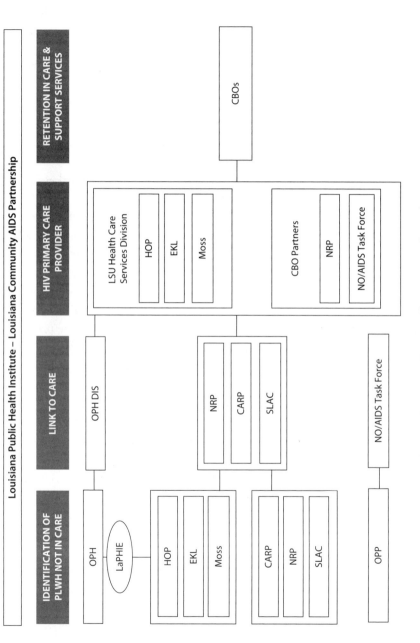

Louisiana Public Health Institute – Louisiana Community AIDS Partnership

| IDENTIFICATION OF PLWH NOT IN CARE | LINK TO CARE | HIV PRIMARY CARE PROVIDER | RETENTION IN CARE & SUPPORT SERVICES |

Figure 1. Louisiana Positive Charge network graphic

figure, the OPH STI/HIV/AIDS Program worked with OPH DIS officers to identify individuals who were in need of linkage-to-care services. The DIS officer worked primarily with PLWH identified through OPH STI clinics, OPH public testing sites, and LaPHIE. The participants were then linked to primary care within the LSU public health system or were linked to care at a CBO that provides HIV primary care.

Health navigators from three CBOs worked with LSU health care providers in New Orleans, Baton Rouge, and Lake Charles to identify PLWH who were out of care. As shown in figure 1, in New Orleans, a health navigator from NRP worked at HOP; in Baton Rouge, a health navigator from CARP worked at EKL; and in Lake Charles, a health navigator from SLAC worked at Moss. The health navigators also relied on LaPHIE to identify out-of-care patients, as represented by the line linking LaPHIE to LSU public hospital (LaPHIE is symbolized by an oval shape since it is a database, not an organization). Health navigators linked their clients to primary care services within the LSU public hospital system or to primary care services provided by their CBO.

Also, a pre/post-release case manager from NO/AIDS Task Force worked with the OPP in New Orleans to link former inmates to HIV medical services after release. The pre/post-release case manager linked clients to the primary care service provider most appropriate for the individual. HIV primary care providers, retention in care, and support services all played a critical and often concurrent role in linkage to primary care and retention in care. PC DIS officers, health navigators, and the pre/post-release case managers linked clients to support services throughout the program, both before and after linkage to primary care. Support services from local CBOs included housing/shelter, mental health services, substance use treatment, benefits assistance, food pantries, and post-incarceration services. Working with support services to address competing needs is an important step in linking clients to care. It is often not until these needs are addressed that clients are ready to focus on their health.

Network Sociogram

Figure 2 is a sociogram of the PC linkage-to-care network in Louisiana. To assess the ties between organizations and the change in ties following PC, we examined the number of ties between organizations using UCINET (Borgatti et al. 2002). Sites were asked whether they had worked with PC partners to link PLWH to care in the six months prior to the start of the project. This allows a pre/post comparison of the network. Figure 2 represents the PC network

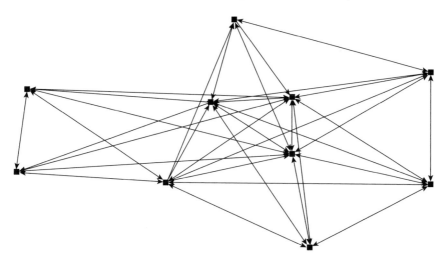

Figure 2. Louisiana Positive Charge network sociogram

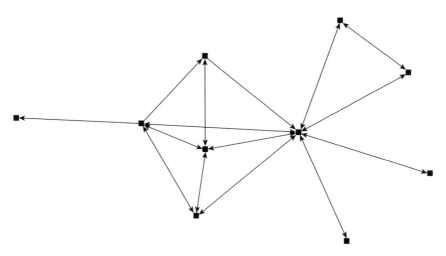

Figure 3. Louisiana organizational network sociogram six months before Positive Charge

following implementation of the project, and figure 3 depicts this information prior to PC.

As shown in figure 2, the density of the Louisiana PC network following implementation was 0.69, meaning that there were 62 out of 90 possible ties. Ties are not necessarily reciprocal; that is, a tie exists when at least one of the two organizations work together. The average degree, or average number of connections per organization, is 6.2. Network centralization, or the extent to which one organization holds the network connections, is moderate for this network at 31%.

In addition to gathering data about the current relationships between Louisiana PC partners, we also asked each site at baseline whether they had worked with their PC partners to link PLWH to care in the six months before the start of the project. This information allowed us to compare the linkage-to-care networks before and after the start of the PC. As figure 3 shows, the linkage-to-care network before PC had a density of 0.30, a total of 27 ties out of 90, and an average degree of 2.7. This network was less dense, included fewer ties, and had a much lower average degree compared with the PC network during project implementation. Network centralization was 69%, which is higher than during PC.

Internal Structural Changes

All organizations reported that PC had positively affected their systems of health care delivery and noted changes to their internal health care delivery systems. One internal structural change was that staff were housed at multiple partner organizations. At HOP, Moss, and EKL, health navigators from CBOs were based in the clinics, and at OPP, a caseworker from NO/AIDS Task Force spent several days a week in the prison. These staff additions constituted major internal structural changes.

Another major change was seen with appointments. One health navigator indicated that he was changing the landscape of what a standard intake appointment looked like. As he explained, "Standard intake was lab visit, social worker visit, and then health education. I am inserting myself into this intake routine so I can talk briefly with HIV clients to make them aware of PC services" (Org. H). At Org. H, the health navigator saw all individuals who were newly diagnosed in the emergency room (ER). This system was not in place before PC. At Org. F, the caseworker from Org. A was embedded within the Org. F medical care system. Org. F made it the standard of care that all incarcerated individuals who were living with HIV met with the PC linkage case manager in Org. F to coordinate linkage-to-care activities on their release from prison. This system did not exist before PC. Another peer navigator explained how he worked with the intake nurse at one of the hospitals to develop a health navigator appointment system:

We tried to develop methods where we were always personally looking for out-of-care patients and then building in appointment systems between us. When we first started, if I was not there, they would just give me their number to contact me, but sometimes we would miss clients. But then we developed, OK we will start doing appointments. They would not be clinic appointments but peer navigator appointments. So if I was out of the office and the intake coordinator at the clinic was speaking to a client who she noticed was out of care or at risk for falling out of care, she would schedule them to come see me. And we started making a referral list from her to me for clients. She sees all new patients at the clinic. —Org. I

Systems for how PLWH are identified have been altered in other ways, as well. For example, at Org. C, before PC, the health educator would periodically go to infection control within the hospital system to determine whether newly diagnosed PLWH who had been referred to care were accessing care. Following PC, the task was being done systematically by the PC health navigator.

Organizations also indicated that they took steps to change the timing of medical appointments. As one respondent explained:

Another thing that contributes to folks falling out of care is that they have so much time between appointments. We had 3 weeks, now it's down to 1.5 to 2 weeks from lab to appointment. Labs on Monday–Thursday don't need appointments, so we stopped making appointments and had the clients come in so they would not have to wait for appointments. We had to look for alternative ways to get things done. —Org. G

Identification of Clients

Effective identification of PLWH who were out of care took close collaboration with partner organizations. Several organizations worked closely with OPH and enrolled participants referred from OPH testing facilities and LSU emergency rooms by DIS officers. These referrals included both newly diagnosed individuals and individuals who had been diagnosed in the past and identified by LaPHIE as not having a recent HIV primary care visit. For example, the DIS officers in New Orleans indicated that they regularly referred clients to Org. I, especially clients without insurance. A health navigator explained:

With the DIS, the disease intervention specialist, through the Office of Public Health, we have really formalized our connection with them in that both [name omitted] and [name omitted] regularly refer their clients straight to us, and know exactly who to call to make sure that the participant has made their appointment, so it is a reality. So instead of just saying go show up at the [Org. I], and not really knowing if they do or don't, it has really firmed up the connection. And the same goes for the [Org. C] linkage in working with [name omitted] the health navigator over there. It works the same way. —Health navigator, Org. I

The health navigator employed by Org. G and stationed at Org. J stated:

I get referrals from [Org. D]; I work closely with DIS officers there. They will have identified someone who has come in for testing at one of their facilities. I also get referrals from [Org. G], from rapid testing there. Referrals come from our own hospital ER and from some of the primary care physicians here as well. —Org. G

In these examples, the health navigators explained how they regularly worked with various PC organizations to identify individuals who were out of care. Respondents also mentioned getting referrals from primary care physicians and from a wide variety of CBOs. In addition, many individuals self-referred into the program after hearing about it from outreach activities or from the network of current participants. Respondents also discussed outreach as a means of identifying out-of-care individuals. Organizations were doing community-based street outreach and outreach at mobile and venue-based HIV testing sites.

Creating out-of-care lists was a strategy employed across most of the sites. These lists allowed identification of individuals who had not been accessing care. For clinical partners, LaPHIE played a key role in identifying PLWH who had been out of care for a certain time, such as one year or six months. Making contact and following up with clients on the out-of-care list required a high level of interorganizational collaboration. For example, Org. B reviewed its client records and identified individuals who were out of care, and then Org. I's health navigator used this list to follow up with out-of-care individuals. Another organization had a list of every patient Org. D had ever referred to them and was therefore able to identify individuals who were referred but did not make an appointment. In addition, organizations were able to use their own internal databases to create lists of out-of-care clients. Respondents stressed the importance of meticulously going through the lists to identify which individuals were truly out of care by cross-checking with external data sources such as lists of incarcerated individuals and death indices. Sites also cross-checked their lists with other databases, such as the ER database or a case management database, to obtain the most up-to-date information, including contact information. Other strategies employed to identify alternative contact information included going through all clinical notes and patient documents.

Outreach and Linkage to Care

To understand the linkage-to-care landscape before the start of PC, we asked each organization to describe how linkage to care was being conducted before the PC program. Most sites had been doing limited linkage-to-care work that was impaired by lack of structure and staffing. For example, a representative from Org. D explained that before PC, the LaPHIE database was used to identify individuals who were out of care, but this information was used only for reporting and statistical purposes. A health educator at Org. C said that, before PC, she would make a small number of calls a week to individuals who were newly diagnosed within the LSU public hospital system to see whether they had been linked to care. However, there was no additional follow-up, and there was no mechanism to identify and link individuals who were previously in care and had dropped out of care. Respondents at multiple organizations mentioned that before PC, they would refer out-of-care individuals to HIV primary care services, but that these referrals were not followed up, were not necessarily tailored to meet the individual needs of their clients, and were most often made to an organization rather than to a specific individual working within the organization. In contrast, Org. A indicated that it had been providing linkage-to-care services as part of its outreach work for many years. Org. G ran a successful medical case management linkage-to-care program before PC, and PC became an extension of this work, allowing the organization to better document and evaluate its linkage-to-care activities.

PC linkage-to-care specialists used a variety of strategies to contact PC participants, including phone calls, home visits, and letters. Sites reiterated that taking the time to fully understand participants' needs and concerns was critical for building rapport and establishing trust. For peers, sharing their own story and listening to the stories of their clients was another important step in building a relationship and establishing credibility. Across all sites, building relationships and addressing barriers to care were key components of linkage to care.

> I do the screener [for needs and barriers to care] and do what I need to do to get them back into care. Whatever the screener tells me then. I make sure they have x, y, z ... Different pieces of the puzzle come out in the screen. I work with them to get what they need. —Org. I

In Louisiana, substance use, housing, and unemployment were the most pressing concerns communicated by PC clients to PC organizations. In addition, many participants faced barriers related to transportation. Some participants needed additional information and education to improve their understanding of why HIV care is important even when one does not feel sick.

Once a participant was ready to be linked to care, PC linkage-to-care workers facilitated the linkage through a variety of strategies, such as making appointments, arranging or providing transportation, giving appointment reminders, and attending lab and clinic appointments. In addition, health navigators helped PC clients to navigate the LSU hospital system by walking them through the screening process and helping them gather the documents they might need, such as ID cards, social security cards, a letter of declaration for individuals who were not employed, and medical records, and ensuring that clients were eligible for free care. The health navigators, DIS officers, and post-release manager continued to work with their clients through phone calls, home visits, provision of transportation, and accompaniment to appointments until barriers to care had been addressed and clients were established in a regular system of care.

Organizations reported that their partnerships with the other PC organizations helped them to better meet the needs of their clients. For example, Org. C and Org. H worked together to implement PC in New Orleans. One organization was located on the East Bank the other on the West Bank. The Org. C / Org. H coordinator could schedule appointments with linkage clients on the East or West Bank, depending on a client's preference. This flexibility reduced the transportation burden placed on clients.

Facilitators of PC Implementation

Several facilitating factors were described by members of the PC network. These included relationships with partner organizations, buy-in from upper-level management, proactive health navigators, and strategically placed incentives.

Relationships with partner organizations

All organizations indicated that having good working relationships with partner organizations was critical to successful linkage of participants to care and treatment. Respondents at several organizations mentioned that they highly valued the support given by the lead agency in overseeing the program. Some commented that, before PC, the organizations involved in the project had operated as separate entities. PC had made them more interested in and aware of the work being done by partner organizations. This awareness helped organizations recognize how they could work together, and having the common goal of linkage to care had facilitated interorganizational collaboration. Other organizations had a long history of working together before the PC program, and this history facilitated a smooth implementation of the program.

Buy-in from upper-level management

Several organizations indicated that the interorganizational collaborations, which are central to PC, would not have been possible without upper management's support and buy-in at partnering organizations. This buy-in was achieved through open and straightforward conversation during the initial planning stages about what each organization needed. By listening to each other and not pushing a preestablished agenda, organizations were able to devise practical programs that met everyone's needs. As a result, partner organizations were heavily invested in the success of the program.

The health navigators also discussed the importance of upper-level management support. For health navigators housed at multiple locations, having someone in a position of authority on their side at each location was important to establishing a smooth transition at the start of the project.

Outgoing, proactive linkage workers

Organizations indicated that having health navigators who were proactive and tenacious was essential to the success of the program. Organizations also highlighted the benefits of having a health navigator who was an advocate for their patients. One supervisor described her organization's health navigator as follows: "Many clients have expressed that if it were not for him [the linkage worker] they would not be in care. Most importantly it [his work] gets a groundwork for establishing that relationship . . . [His] efforts exceed all expectations" (Org. I).

Incentives

Respondents at multiple organizations mentioned that an incentive for the first medical visit boosted attendance. Incentives were often store gift cards in $10 or $20 increments.

Unmet Client Needs and Barriers to PC Implementation

Organizations faced many barriers to PC implementation. A variety of challenges were discussed during the in-depth interviews with program staff, including interorganizational collaboration, providers' and clients' attitudes about HIV, and resource or structural issues and unmet needs.

Interorganizational Collaboration
Integration into the public hospital system

In Louisiana, the PC health navigators from local CBOs spent much of their time in the public hospitals. It took time for the health navigators to feel integrated into the public hospital system. One barrier to integration was that while upper management had detailed knowledge about the program, some of the other medical staff were not clear about the role of the health navigators and the distinction between a health navigator and a social worker. This confusion initially hindered collaboration. As a health navigator explained, "Folks knew I was coming, but they did not know much about who I was or my role. The director and key supervisors knew, but I am not certain that the other staff was too aware" (employee of Org. H stationed at Org. C). Another health navigator noted:

> At first medical providers didn't understand what I was providing nor did they want to know. I have a hospital badge so why am I being treated like this? Said, can I please speak to you in private whenever you have time, and then I would just talk to them individually one on one. Explained why I needed to come to the hospital and why I couldn't just be stationary. A few made referrals to me of family members, well that broke the barrier right there.   Employee of Org. G stationed at Org. J

In addition, initial linkage-to-care data demonstrated to medical staff the positive impact that health navigators were having on their clients living with HIV. Sharing these data helped hospital staff to understand the work of the health navigators better and to recognize and value their contribution.

While staff hoped to conduct trainings for medical staff on health navigation, scheduling proved challenging. Instead, health navigators educated medical staff about health navigation at the clinics, through brief, brown bag presentations and one-on-one conversations. Health navigators also worked with staff to integrate health navigation into existing hospital systems.

Office logistics

Several organizations indicated that finding office space for the health navigators had been a challenge. Organizations also faced challenges in working with partner organizations to ensure that health navigators had access to the necessary office equipment, such as a phone and a computer.

Contacting people who were out of care

Linkage workers repeatedly said that making the initial contact with individuals who were out of care was extremely difficult. Most sites used preexisting medical health records that included basic demographic information, contact information, and an emergency contact. Relying on cellphones to reach people was not feasible because cellphone numbers change frequently, clients often lacked minutes, or phones were turned off. Given that staying in contact with participants is a key aspect of linkage-to-care work, sites suggested offering participants unlimited cellphone minutes as an incentive to stay in the program and increase ease of contact.

Attitudinal Barriers
Attitudes of hospital staff

Another barrier was that some hospital staff did not understand why such an emphasis was being placed on HIV. An administrator explained:

> We have been instrumental in changing the attitudes of providers at the hospital. Since HIV is an infectious disease there is an urgency to get people into care, but there was resistance. Why are these people getting so much special treatment, if they are not in care that is their problem. But I know that if they had a bad experience in the ER or lab or screening they are not going to come back. —Employee of Org. G stationed at Org. J

Client reticence toward HIV care

Some out-of-care individuals were resistant to entering or reentering the HIV care system. Working with participants required a significant time commitment and a high level of attention. When working with clients, health navigators focused first on building the relationship, and once this relationship was established, in some instances, they were able to start discussions about HIV care and treatment. As one health navigator said, "I really try to . . . develop a bit of a relationship with them, tell them a bit of my story. That I am working for them. Then after that, some feel comfortable and will want to move ahead" (Org. I).

Resource and Structural Issues and Unmet Needs
Competing needs / shortage of support services

Another challenge was that linkage workers found that before linking someone to care, they had to identify and address the issues keeping the individual from accessing care. This process could be time consuming, and the resources needed to address these barriers were not always available or appropriate for participants. Organizations indicated a shortage in a variety of support services for PLWH, including mental health treatment, substance use treatment, job placement, and housing. For example, Org. G estimated that somewhere between 45% and 55% of their clients had both mental health and substance use disorders and that there was a dearth of services to address these needs. A health navigator at Org. H indicated that a lot of their clients were homeless or unstably housed. While some housing services were available for their clients, there were long turnaround times, and many of the available services were for group living, which was often not appealing for clients. Linkage workers indicated that it can take months to get a client into housing and, during this time, it is easy to lose contact. The PC post-release case manager who worked with incarcerated populations noted that housing was the number one concern for most individuals who were coming out of jail.

Linkage workers also indicated a need for job placement programs. Many of their clients were on a low income or had no income. One linkage worker knew of only one job placement program, and it had very slow placement. He expressed the need for services to help his clients find safe employment opportunities.

Centralized services

Sites reported the need for more centralized services for PLWH.

> One of the reasons our clients fall out of care is because we have them going all over the place. They have to go here for this, or they have to go there for food.

And they don't have the transportation . . . it is like pulling teeth to get them in the door and then you tell them to leave, to go over there to get that. —Org. I

Transportation

Regardless of their location, organizations reported that for many of their clients, transportation was a barrier to HIV care and treatment. In Louisiana, a lack of access to affordable and efficient transportation affected the ability of PLWH to access care and remain in care. For example, for sites in Lake Charles, public transportation is limited within the city and runs only until 6 pm. Outside the city, no public transportation is available. Participants also reported that Medicaid transportation was not reliable.

Clients' need for medications to treat conditions other than HIV

Due to funding limitations, Louisiana's medication assistance program from Ryan White Part B funding was eliminated. PC sites found that this adversely affected clients who were taking medication, primarily for mental health issues, diabetes, or high cholesterol.

Staffing needs

Sites also noted the need for additional retention-in-care staff to work with individuals who were not out of care. They stated that if there were more resources to focus on retaining folks in care, this would reduce the number of PLWH who dropped out of care and potentially reduce the workload associated with locating and reestablishing care for people who had fallen out of care. Some sites indicated the need for additional staff to support data collection activities, including data entry, data monitoring, and data analysis.

Policy

When asked about policy, several respondents at PC sites had difficulty articulating how policy affects their work with PLWH. Others responded about policy across various levels, including federal, state, and organization policy. Several sites mentioned ADAP, waitlists, and the need for more funding for HIV medication. Individuals who worked with incarcerated populations expressed frustration that they were not able to begin the application processes for social support services such as housing until after the individual was released. This process caused considerable delays in getting someone stably housed and made it more challenging to link someone to care after release.

Another site expressed frustration that state-level HIV policy was mandated without proper thought or resources given to ensure the policy was appropriately implemented. Some respondents also mentioned that policies were needed to make it easier for Louisiana residents to get state identification cards, because state IDs are necessary to receive care at state hospitals. Getting an ID can take time and be burdensome, which can delay entry and reentry into care.

Overarching Conclusions

After implementation of the PC program at the Louisiana sites, partner organizations formed measurably closer working relationships, including housing staff at each other's organizations. These collaborations strongly enhanced client identification and linkage to care in a variety of ways, including co-development of lists of out-of-care clients. Clients were better served because the services provided could be tailored to their specific situations. This process was helped by management-level staff's understanding of partner organizations' needs. Interorganizational challenges reported by many health navigators included confusion about their role and insufficient resources to accommodate them at their home organization (e.g., a phone and a computer). This issue was addressed mainly through open communication between frontline staff across organizations. Future programs may enhance collaboration by fostering this type of cross-organizational communication.

Chicago

Background

As of June 2013, there were 16,538 people living with HIV (PLWH) and 18,608 people living with AIDS in Chicago, including 691 HIV cases diagnosed from January to June of 2013 and 454 AIDS cases in this time period (Illinois Department of Public Health [IDPH] 2013). As seen nationally, Black/African Americans accounted for a disproportionately large share of the HIV and AIDS epidemic in Chicago (IDPH 2013). While representing only 33% of the Chicago population, Black/African Americans comprised more than half (51.1%) of HIV cases in Chicago since 2006 (U.S. Census Bureau 2010a; IDPH 2013). Of all HIV diagnoses since 2006, 24% were among Caucasians, 17% among Latinos, and 6% among other races/ethnicities. Almost 80% of PLWH diagnosed since 2006 were men. In 2013, men who have sex with men was the mode of exposure for 51% of HIV transmissions across all racial/ethnic groups (IDPH 2013).

Illinois received $124,944,075 in federal HIV and AIDS grant funding in FY 2013. The largest proportion was Ryan White HIV/AIDS Program funding ($85,038,961), followed by Centers for Disease Control and Prevention HIV funding ($24,249,937) and funding from Housing Opportunities for Persons with AIDS ($9,289,916), Substance Abuse and Mental Health Services Administration ($6,023,887), and Office of Minority Health HIV and AIDS ($341,374) (Kaiser Family Foundation 2012). The total AIDS Drug Assistance Program (ADAP) budget for Illinois for FY 2012 was $60,787,759, a 16% increase from FY 2011. As of June 2013, 8,610 clients were enrolled in ADAP (NASTAD 2014).

Program Overview

Project Identify, Navigate, Connect, Access, Retain, and Evaluate (IN-CARE) was a multiagency, multifaceted intervention model that aimed to facilitate access to and retention in care for men who have sex with men (MSM) living with HIV in Chicago. Project IN-CARE, led by the AIDS Foundation of Chicago (AFC), was a collaboration between diverse nonprofit organizations involved in HIV testing, case management, and medical services for adult men living with HIV at risk of delayed or interrupted care access in the Chicago area. The project used standard care practices along with innovative health interventions such as peer health navigation and group-based HIV education.

Project IN-CARE was a partnership of two clinical organizations and a community-based organization that, as described by one participant, had "the goal of identifying people who are newly diagnosed or lost to care, navigating them through the service system, connecting them to necessary services, whether that be case management, housing, etc., assessing barriers to care and helping individuals identify ways to overcome some of those barriers to care, retaining people in primary care for at least the nine-month period if not longer, and then evaluating the effectiveness of the patient health navigation" (Org. A). AFC funded local organizations to provide direct services. The three IN-CARE organizations offered a variety of services, but all offered similar peer services. AFC served as the peers' point of contact for questions related to participant enrollment and supported the subcontracted organizations in their assessments.

The six components of the proposed Project IN-CARE were innovations to **I**dentify and enroll MSM living with HIV at risk of interruption of or nonadherence to care; to provide short-term peer health **N**avigation for newly diagnosed or out-of-care men; to **C**onnect men to care through HIV case management; to facilitate **A**ccess to primary care, lab services, and medications through existing medical and social services; to enhance **R**etention of participants in care through an eighteen-hour, peer-led, group-based education system; and to **E**valuate the effectiveness of the program.

Positive Charge Partner Organizations

The Positive Charge (PC) network in Chicago was made up of four nonprofit organizations, as outlined below.

1. *AIDS Foundation of Chicago (AFC)*: AFC is a foundation that works with community organizations to develop and improve services for PLWH, funds and coordinates HIV prevention and care programs, and advocates for HIV policy. The foundation manages more than $17 million in local, state, and federal funds for an array of HIV-related services, including case management, housing, and nutrition. As the lead agency in the Positive Charge network, AFC oversaw and coordinated PC activities.

2. *Test Positive Aware Network (TPAN):* TPAN is a community-based organization that offers a variety of integrated services. Its services include prevention outreach, intake assessment, information and referral services, HIV counseling and testing, needle exchange, hepatitis / sexually transmitted infection (STI) screening, clinical services, alternative therapies, case management, treatment education, psychosocial support, substance use services, and information dissemination. In the context of Positive Charge, TPAN implemented activities to link clients to and retain them in care.

3. *Ruth M. Rothstein CORE Center:* The CORE Center is a health clinic that focuses on prevention, care, and research for HIV, AIDS, and other infectious diseases in the Chicago area. It was founded in 1998. The center has a "one-stop shop" model, aiming to provide clients with a full array of health and social services at one location. The services offered include primary and specialty medical care, dental care, social support services, prevention and education programs, confidential testing and treatment for STIs, HIV, and tuberculosis, and research. The CORE Center contributed to PC by providing clients with services, and health navigators assisted clients in accessing these services and linkage to care.

4. *Howard Brown Health Center (HBHC):* HBHC is a health and social service delivery organization that serves lesbian, gay, bisexual, and transgender individuals. The health center, founded in 1974, has seven divisions: primary medical care, behavioral health, research, HIV/STI prevention, youth services, elder services, and community initiatives. It also offers services related to HIV and AIDS, including medical services, case management, counseling, psychotherapy, programs for young PLWH, group therapy, workshops, and support groups. HIV medical services include general check-ups, medication monitoring and management, coordination of counseling and social services, specialty referrals, therapies such as acupuncture, chiropractic care, massage, and nutrition services.

HBHC's annual budget exceeds $22 million, and the center serves more than 36,000 adults and youth per year. The center has three service-delivery locations: the main health and research center in Uptown, the Broadway Youth Center, and the Triad Health Practice in the Advocate Illinois Masonic Medical Center. As part of the PC program, health navigators based at HBHC assisted clients in accessing its services and linkage to care.

Tables 5 and 6 summarize the characteristics of these PC sites and the services they provided to clients.

Table 5 Positive Charge network partners, Chicago

Organization	Legal fiscal designation	Type of health service agency	Annual HIV operation budget	Number of PLWH served, 2010	Number of paid employees, 2010	Number of volunteers, 2010
AIDS Foundation of Chicago (AFC)	Private nonprofit	Advocacy and service coordination agency	~$19 million	~5,500	~70	100+
Test Positive Aware Network (TPAN)	Private nonprofit	HIV and AIDS service organization	$2.6 million	550	35	40
Ruth M. Rothstein CORE Center	Public	Hospital-based clinic	$20 million (overall)	~6,000	250	0
Howard Brown Health Center (HBHC)	Private nonprofit	Community-based organization	~$15 million (overall in 2010)	1,500	264*	175*

*Information from Form 990 (HBHC 2010).

Table 6 Services offered to PLWH by PC partner organizations, Chicago

Organization	STI/HIV counseling and testing	HIV primary care	HIV case management	HIV outreach and linkage to care	HIV peer support	Other health services	Counseling services	HIV education and prevention services	Assistance with entitlement services	Support services*
AIDS Foundation of Chicago (AFC)	×		×	×	×	×	×	×	×	H, T, N, S
Test Positive Aware Network (TPAN)	×		×	×	×	×	×	×	×	H, S
Ruth M. Rothstein CORE Center	×	×	×	×	×	×	×	×	×	H, N, S
Howard Brown Health Center (HBHC)	×	×	×	×	×	×	×	×	×	T, N, S

*H = housing; N = nutritional support or food; S = substance use treatment; T = transportation.

Chicago Positive Charge Network
Network Graphic

Figure 4 represents the Chicago PC network. Organizations are represented by boxes. The gray boxes at the top indicate the role of each organization in the linkage-to-care continuum. For Project IN-CARE, this continuum includes identification of PLWH who are out of care, outreach and linkage to care, provision of HIV primary care, and retention in care and support services. As represented by the long box at the top of the figure, AFC was the lead agency for Project IN-CARE and oversaw and coordinated PC linkage-to-care activities in Chicago.

Linkage-to-care activities were implemented by three IN-CARE partner organizations: TPAN, CORE Center, and HBHC. Starting at the top left corner of the figure, the line between the "Community-based clinics" and "TPAN" boxes represents collaboration between TPAN and a variety of community-based clinics that provided HIV and STI testing services. Specifically, TPAN's peer health navigator conducted outreach at community-based testing clinics and received referrals from these clinics. The peer health navigator then worked with a variety of HIV primary care providers to link individuals to care, including Cook County Ambulatory Primary Care, CORE Center, HBHC, and other primary care providers. In contrast, at CORE Center and HBHC, most of the identification of out-of-care PLWH, outreach and linkage, provision of primary care, and provision of support services occurred under one roof. At both CORE and HBHC, peers assisted PLWH in navigating the range of services offered by these "one-stop shops."

As indicated in figure 4 by the lines connecting the boxes under "HIV Primary Care Provider" to those under "Retention in Care & Support Services," all of IN-CARE's peer health navigators linked participants to retention-in-care services and to support services. Each of the three IN-CARE implementing partner organizations provided retention and self-management services in-house. In addition, IN-CARE participants were referred to agencies such as the Northeastern Illinois Case Management Cooperative. IN-CARE peer navigators worked with a variety of support service organizations to meet the ongoing housing, mental health, and substance use needs of their clients. IN-CARE peers worked with approximately twelve agencies that provided housing services, fifteen that provided mental health services, and fifteen that provided substance use services.

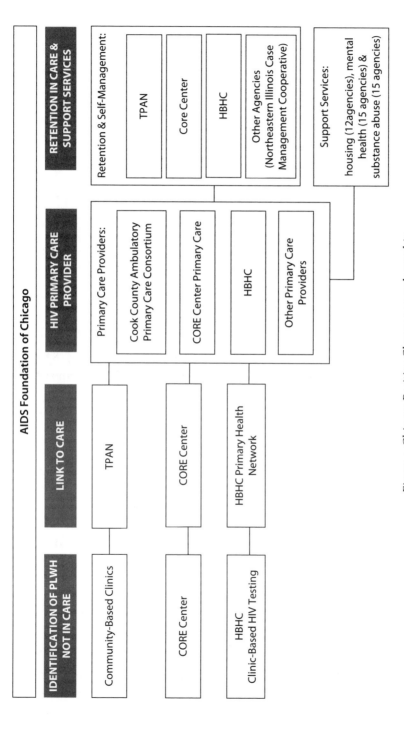

Figure 4. Chicago Positive Charge network graphic

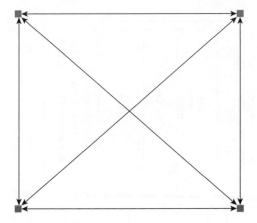

Figure 5. Chicago organizational network sociogram during and six months before Positive Charge

Network Sociogram

We assessed the ties among organizations and the change in these ties following implementation of PC, using UCINET (Borgatti et al. 2002). Sites were asked which PC partners they worked with during the PC project and whether they had worked with these partners to link PLWH to care in the six months before the project. These two questions allowed a comparison between the linkage-to-care networks before and after the start of PC.

Figure 5 is a sociogram of the PC linkage-to-care network in Chicago. Following PC, the Chicago network had a density of 1.0 because all the organizations in the network were linked to one another. This density represents a tightly connected network in which all possible ties among organizations existed. The network included a total of twelve ties. The average degree, or number of connections per organization, is 3. The network centralization is 0%, meaning that all organizations were equally connected to the others. Before PC, the sociogram was the same: Chicago's network had a density of 1, and the network centralization was 0%.

Internal Structural Changes

No large staff changes were associated with the implementation of Project IN-CARE, but there were some shifts in priorities within the organizations. Rather than creating new structures or new relationships among partners, the existing systems were adapted to implement the new Project IN-CARE model. For example, one organization explained how the project helped it prioritize evaluation:

The value of evaluation, the value of the data, I think really . . . hit home around the time that we got this grant . . . I mean definitely, you know, we do know now we have these 300 people and we have all of this rich data that we can use to develop programs. You know, we also have case management data as well, but having a team that actually takes the time to do some of that analysis, to do some of that review, I think has been really invaluable and really helpful and really sort of came about from this project and this project having such a rigorous evaluation. —Org. A

The use of peer navigators in IN-CARE was seen as a mechanism for reducing the workload of overburdened case managers:

Being one of the agencies that host the IN-CARE project, for us it's been—I kind of refer to it as case management light, like case management for people who don't really need a full case manager. It helps resolve the issue of overloading case managers, and most of the clients we see don't need the full benefits of a case manager, even though some think they do. So this is a way of alleviating a lot of work from our case managers and other organizations' case managers. —Org. B

Implementation agencies described some structural changes during Project IN-CARE. These included, at one organization, personnel shifts in which different individuals took over responsibility for administration of the project and peer navigation and, at another, the hiring of an additional navigator. One organization also began using touch-screen tablets during the project so that the testing team and linkage-to-care team could immediately schedule appointments.

Identification of Clients

Respondents described various mechanisms to identify individuals who were eligible for Project IN-CARE. Some of the organizations had active outreach and HIV testing programs. They also identified individuals when they came in for STI testing: "Ideally, what brings them in is they want to be tested for an STI, but because we do everything, including hepatitis screening, they get their HIV test done also. If [at] that point, if they are positive, they get the results that day" (Org. C). Organizations that did not provide their own HIV testing services, however, struggled to identify individuals who were eligible for Project IN-CARE. Eventually, one organization was able to develop effective network-based and online mechanisms for identifying participants:

> Our first successful project was doing it online . . . this was kind of developing a piece where we had a presence in various chat rooms from across the city and just with an introduction as to who we were and then an invitation into getting more information. And from there we would invite people into the agency and kind of go through the recruitment process . . . an even better way was identifying the few enrolled clients into IN-CARE as being what I call agents. And these agents are incentivized to go out and bring in people that fit the criteria. And that was just really, really successful. —Org. B

Outreach and Linkage to Care

Interviewees described the value of the outreach and linkage components of Project IN-CARE. Previously, the organizations had relied on informal provider and organizational networks, but IN-CARE "was the first sort of concerted effort to really identify and link newly diagnosed [individuals] to a different kind of an intervention as well as trying to identify folks who may have dropped out of care with a very sort of defined intervention" (Org. A).

A number of active processes were used to link recently diagnosed individuals to care immediately. At one organization, recently diagnosed PLWH were introduced to a navigator on the same day that they were tested and were scheduled for a follow-up appointment. This was done to ensure that people who were newly diagnosed did not leave before they were connected to the clinic and to a peer educator or navigator. The navigator later called the individuals who were newly diagnosed to check on how they were doing and to remind them of upcoming appointments. The navigator stayed with the individuals during their entire first care visit and worked with them to address potential barriers and challenges that they might face:

> So they walk them through, they stay with them until they literally kind of walk out the door. At that time, there's a conversation about barriers, identifying anyone, [identifying] barriers. There is a conversation about transportation. Can they make sure they get back here? What do we need to do to get you here? If they need bus transportation, of course they get that. If they're like really, really depressed, we hook them up with mental health [services], so we

make sure that the person, the entire person, is taken care of before they walk out the door, so whatever that entails. If that entails meeting someone in chemical dependency [services], that's taken care of. —Org. C

The navigator is invaluable in making PLWH feel okay on that first care visit; "when they come in in that two weeks, they're not alone 'cause this is a huge building. When you walk in, you just don't know anything, but to see someone actually meet you when you come in means the world to someone" (Org. C).

Organizations also attempted to actively monitor PLWH lost to services, using provider referrals to give them additional support, including cab fare. "Whatever reason that stopped them from coming, we need to identify that barrier and we get them to care" (Org. C). This monitoring was sometimes done through an outreach team or through peer navigators who actively followed up with emergency contacts and visited individuals' old addresses to try to find them and bring them back into care. One organization did not have sufficient personnel to review its records for PLWH who were not retained in care. It did, however, get referrals from care providers of individuals who had missed two or more appointments.

Facilitators of PC Implementation

One of the key facilitators for implementation of Project IN-CARE was the strong collaboration and buy-in by the various agencies. Partners were contacted during the proposal-writing process, and all agreed on the importance of linkage to care: "communicating with all of the partners and you know making sure that they all feel connected; that they all feel that they were part of the system . . . helped sort of get this rolling, get this off the ground" (Org. A). It was noted, however, that there should have been more initial engagement with care providers and hospitals.

Strong and capable staff have also helped the agencies surmount the challenges that they faced during implementation of Project IN-CARE. One navigator described the key enablers of the services: "Compassion, knowledge, and I would say time. You give time. They give you all time, don't try to rush patients and clients because you play two games if you're rushing the person: you can't do the good work, or you lose the patient" (Org. D). Navigators also described the importance of a supportive environment in enabling them to deal with the emotional burden of their work. It was also important for agencies to have a lot of different referral and service options available to help clients meet their various needs.

Another key resource for Project IN-CARE was the data collection system. This system allowed the project to identify when individuals had multiple peers so that it could reduce duplication of efforts. The database also enabled Org. A to advocate for peers to spend more time working on tasks specifically related to Project IN-CARE and helped Org. A to identify key areas for intervention. "So a lot of our programming now is becoming less informed by 'I have a hunch that' and more that we found in this program" (Org. A). Additionally, the client intake system provided a mechanism for peers to get to know clients:

> Every client is different. That's what I really like about the program, that I don't think I have any two clients that are the same. I mean, they may have similar needs but there's different ways I may approach them depending on the clients. And the intake and actually the questions and things like that allows me to get to know them better. —Org. B.

Unmet Client Needs and Barriers to PC Implementation

Despite its various successes, Project IN-CARE did have some challenges with recruitment, intervention components, and organizational partnerships. Originally conceptualized to provide care exclusively to men of color, the project "expanded enrollment to include non–men of color in order to increase the enrollment numbers" (Org. A). One proposed component that was not implemented was the online Chronic Care Self-Management Program, which failed to get sufficient funding and thus was not functional.

Project IN-CARE was originally conceived to have two clinic partners and two community-based partners, but one of the sites was ultimately dropped. This site had low recruitment and high turnover. The setback was attributed to a failure to assess the organization's readiness before starting. The organization also had very little experience with provision of direct services.

The peer component of IN-CARE was a central piece of the program, but there were some challenges, including competing work demands for the peers' time and some resistance from case managers who felt threatened by the peers. This case manager resistance "manifested itself initially in the first probably four or five months of the project [in] not returning phone calls, not responding, being sort of rude to the peers on the phone, requesting what I would consider odious amounts of documentation and stuff" (Org. A). The resistance was partially related to lack of clarity about task allocation, such as who gave participants their bus passes. In response to this resistance, the lead agency organized a mandatory meeting with all of the case managers and peers. At this meeting, they

> basically sort of really set the boundary for what the two [case managers and peers] were going to be doing and what the difference was between the two, and I think, and it's not to say that it cleared it all up and it was all kumbayah afterwards, but I think it was at least good for the case managers to see that the goal[s] of these peer positions are really to support overburdened case managers to get people connected to care and to provide them with resources and support that they [case managers] may not be able to do. —Org. A

Peer navigators also dealt with this resistance on a one-on-one basis:

> I had to basically meet with the case managers and explain the program, explain to them that it's not meant to take over case management. It's meant to complement them [case managers]. And I let them know my boundaries, my limits and things that I could do. That they're basically still doing their job and they still have their position and their signature would go a whole lot further than my signature. And to let them know that if they need basically some assistance or grunt work, if you will, or just need for me to make sure that the client makes the appointments, [or need me to] make the calls to remind the clients or go pick up the clients and kind of escort and go with them to make it easier and more comfortable for the client that they have someone there for support . . . I'm willing to do that, and I'm able to do that, time willing. —Org. B

Some navigators did feel frustrated with their narrowly defined tasks and inability to make referrals to help their clients: "Let us help our clients to the best of our ability. Don't tie our hands up" (Org. C). Also, there were some logistical challenges for navigators. It was challenging for entry-level navigators to manage all of the data collection and processing because they did not have computer skills. As a result, one organizational administrator suggested that navigators should have computer training before the start of the project. They also underscored the need for additional navigators, particularly for larger organizations.

Despite the formal connections among organizations through Project IN-CARE, project staff explained that they primarily worked in isolation and had little communication from the project administrators. One administrator felt that the IN-CARE system in which clients could be with only one organization made collaboration seem "contraindicated." Another administrator felt that it might be beneficial for organizations to collaborate more:

> I think we have isolated projects. We definitely see more clients here at [Org. C]. It would be nice probably to see them more often just to find out what's working, what's going on at their sites. Certainly more than maybe the steering committee. I would say, probably, maybe one time a month just to get together maybe informally, just to find out what's going on. That would be nice. —Org. C

Respondents also noted challenges and competition in working with other agencies. Respondents from one agency mentioned that none of the clinics were interested in their support and would tell them:

> "We just really don't have the time to do this," or, "We already have something like that in place." And we continue to be like, "No, we're here to help. We're not trying to take your work away from you; we want to help you do your work better." —Org. B

This underscored the need to have "MoUs [memoranda of understanding] with doctors or clinics, even case management staff, [so they can] help identify people—some of their clients—who feel that working with a peer could benefit them" (Org. B).

There was a gap in staffing at the lead agency due to a medical leave, and some partners felt disconnected: "When someone's out sick, we don't hear anything, but just [that] the person's out sick. Don't know where to send information to" (Org. C). The lead agency did learn from that experience, however, and developed a back-up system. One organization thought that the lead agency had fulfilled its job well:

> They have been the most supportive. It's not my first time to work for [Org. A], the most supportive, the most organized, the most open to hearing our struggles and our successes, so congratulatory around the successes. I can't think of anything that I would want [done] differently than what they've done for us. —Org B

Participants provided constructive feedback to the lead agency on enhancing its communication with partners. During a time when a key project leader had an extended absence, the break in communications proved problematic. Participants also frequently mentioned challenges presented by the paperwork system. Lack of Spanish-language materials (described on the next page) was a key challenge, as was the confusing nature of some of the questions: "Some of the clients really don't understand some of the questions. Some of the clients may feel that they're too personal, which I always let them know that, you know, if anything's too personal we could stop or you could just skip it or something like that" (Org. B).

Some participants also thought that the definition of "out-of-care" for eligibility was problematic because some individuals who were nonadherent were not eligible for the program:

> Usually, if someone is HIV-positive they're supposed to see a doctor every three months, three to four months. If the client's only seen a doctor twice in the year, meaning they missed two medical appointments . . . in my opinion that person would not be in care, or just because the person went to the doctor and got blood work that does not mean they're taking their medications. So that person would not be in care. So I think more information should be added to the eligibility question, to open it up to people who technically are not in care, instead of just going by medical visits . . . I would add the missed visits, the medication adherence. Substance abuse could be one of the criteria. And just their mental status. —Org. B

A central unmet need noted by organizations was for more communication between the various agencies and stronger collaboration. Similarly, one peer navigator emphasized the need for networking and stronger referrals among agencies: "We cannot talk about people with HIV as 'our' clients. They don't belong to us. Because we can't as an agency provide all the services and reach all their needs. We need to work in the networking" (Org. D). In addition to the desire for more collaboration across organizations within Chicago, one administrator thought that it would be helpful to have opportunities for clients to meet one another and network and to have different PC organizations speak to one another across cities to share ideas and challenges.

One persistent challenge for Project IN-CARE partners was that the agencies had different databases that were not completely compatible, which meant that peers sometimes had to enter the same data twice. The partners hoped to adapt the existing databases so that they could ultimately have one database. Organizations also highlighted a need for additional peers and emphasized that peers should be paid employees of an organization rather than receiving a stipend. Navigators emphasized the need for more training in all areas, not only in computers and working with data.

Respondents consistently expressed an urgent need for documents in Spanish. They all employed Spanish-speaking peers, but translation of documents, including those that were supposed to be self-completed by clients, took a lot of time and affected the quality of participants' responses: "We don't have the whole interview in Spanish [and it] is so difficult. I speak Spanish perfectly . . . You need to translate to that person [to] get the idea [of] what is a question and what is a statement" (Org. C).

In addition to these institutional challenges, a key unmet need for men living with HIV was access to "clean, decent, affordable housing" (Org. A). Participants consistently reported that lack of housing was the biggest challenge facing their clients, and there were also some reports of the need for more transportation.

Policy

The most frequently mentioned policy challenge was the uncertainty about anticipated policy shifts and lack of funding. When asked about the impact of policy at the programmatic level, a respondent at one organization explained that the uncertainty regarding the direction of policy had led to some organizational mandate drift:

> It seems like such an . . . uncertain time . . . I mean, it's changing organizations; it's changing how they define themselves, and it's changing their services . . . and people are doing that to chase the money . . . it makes sense, because they want to stay alive, they want to stay viable, but they aren't necessarily having the conversation about how does that impact who they serve and who they're going to serve. You know, because, like a lot of organizations are, like, we're chronic care now, we're not just HIV. Well, what does that mean in terms of availability of resources for people living with HIV? —Org. A

This respondent underscored the need to inform agencies about impending changes to programs such as Ryan White so that they could appropriately prepare their clients.

Overarching Conclusions

The Chicago PC network was characterized by a tightly connected group of organizations. However, there were some challenges in collaboration: an initial implementation partner had to be dropped from the project, and it was difficult to gain clinical partners. Many interviewees expressed a desire for more collaboration across organizations.

Other challenges included the lack of Spanish-language materials. Recruitment also proved more challenging than expected: the project initially focused on men of color, but too few enrolled, and the program population was expanded to include other groups.

Despite initial resistance, case managers had more manageable workloads as a result of peer navigators' help. The early resistance was addressed through meetings and one-on-one communication. Project administrators also discussed how the increased use and understanding of evaluation allowed case managers and peers to track clients better. Overall, despite some barriers and challenges to implementation, respondents valued Project IN-CARE. They felt that they could better identify the needs of MSM living with HIV in Chicago and enhance their linkage to and retention in care:

> I just want to reiterate again how successful this project has been for us and the really—the good—the good that it's brought to our clients and the agency itself, and it's certainly been a very, very worthy undertaking for us. —Org. B

One respondent described how he could have benefited from similar work in the past:

> I mean, me, if somebody would've came and helped me out long time ago, maybe I wouldn't have lived the homeless life, because I lived the homeless life because of my status, my drug of choice, my lifestyle, everything that was going on. I was a young man. I didn't know . . . I mean, I didn't know . . . But I hung in there. And I know for a fact, again, I've experienced that, [this project] would've meant a lot to me. That would've meant a lot. —Chicago PC network

New York City

Background

New York City had the highest number of diagnosed HIV infections in the United States at the end of 2010, even when compared with other heavily affected metropolitan areas such as Los Angeles, Chicago, Miami, and San Francisco (Centers for Disease Control and Prevention 2011a). Among all U.S. metropolitan statistical areas in 2011, NYC had the ninth-highest rate of HIV infection. During 2012, 3,141 new HIV cases and 1,889 new AIDS cases were diagnosed in NYC; of these, 612 were simultaneous HIV and AIDS diagnoses. Although the number of new infections in NYC is decreasing, the number of people living with HIV (PLWH) is growing. In 2012, there were 114,926 individuals living with HIV or AIDS, and of these individuals, 58.5% had an AIDS diagnosis (New York City Department of Health and Mental Hygiene 2012).

There were significant socioeconomic disparities among those newly diagnosed with HIV. Of the 3,141 individuals newly diagnosed with HIV in 2012, 79.4% were male, 44.4% were Black/African American, and 32.4% were Hispanic. White individuals accounted for 19.5% of new infections (New York City Department of Health and Mental Hygiene 2012). Only 25.5% of NYC's population identifies as Black/African American; 28.6% identify as Hispanic or Latino (U.S. Census Bureau 2010b). Most newly infected individuals resided in low-income NYC zip codes. Specifically, 52% of individuals newly diagnosed with HIV in 2012 lived in areas where 20% or more of the population had an income below the federal poverty line. Not only did poorer neighborhoods have more HIV infections, but individuals living with HIV residing in these neighborhoods had worse long-term health outcomes than their counterparts in other neighborhoods. This disparity in survival rates persists when examining race outside the neighborhood context: individuals of color living with HIV did not survive as long as their White counterparts (New York City Department of Health and Mental Hygiene 2012).

In FY 2012, the State of New York received almost $0.5 billion in federal funding for HIV and AIDS. The majority was through Ryan White funding at $334,774,397. Centers for Disease Control and Prevention funding accounted for $85,502,989, while Housing Opportunities for Persons with AIDS provided $60,548,848. The Substance Abuse and Mental Health Services Administration provided $18,145,138, and the Office of Minority Health contributed $929,921 (Kaiser Family Foundation 2012).

Program Overview

ACCESS NY, the Positive Charge (PC) project in New York City, served low-income PLWH in the five boroughs. It was a two-part project that combined improving access to primary medical care for Medicaid-eligible PLWH who were not receiving treatment and strengthening clinical service systems to retain clients in care. ACCESS NY provided primary care and other services needed by out-of-care individuals (e.g., housing, clothing, meals, legal support, and drugs and alcohol detoxification and rehabilitation).

At the time of the PC project, there were six community health outreach workers (CHOWs) and seven health navigators who worked collaboratively to identify, link, and retain PLWH through the ACCESS NY project. CHOWs were peers who played a more intensive, short-term role in identifying and connecting with potential clients and linking them with resources and health navigators. Health navigators, in turn, filled a more long-term role, providing and connecting clients with medical and social support.

The Learning Collaborative, led by Primary Care Development Corporation (PCDC), was a series of six Learning Sessions in which ACCESS NY clinical partners worked to improve their clients' retention and shared experiences and solutions with other participating centers. The ultimate aim of the Learning Collaborative was to increase access, continuity, and efficiency in each of the participating clinical organizations to ensure that clients could have timely access to care with their provider. Some sites offered same-day appointments. A PCDC staff member was assigned as a coach to each partner organization. Coaches met with leadership at the partner organizations and provided guidance in setting up a change team to improve clinical practices. Change teams were composed of front-desk staff, medical assistants, providers, nurses, and leadership. Learning Sessions were held every two to six months. Participating organizations shared what they had learned and acted as each other's co-consultants.

Positive Charge Partner Organizations

ACCESS NY was a consortium consisting of three key collaborators: New York City AIDS Fund of the New York Community Trust (the Trust), Amida Care, and PCDC. The Trust, the lead organization, provided ongoing management and oversight. Amida Care is a Medicaid Special Needs Plan, and PCDC led the Learning Collaborative. The network also had seven primary care provider partners: Housing Works, HELP PSI / Project Samaritan, Harlem United, Callen-Lorde, Village Care of New York, St. Mary's Episcopal Center, and Acacia Network. With the exception of Callen-Lorde, these primary care providers were sponsor sites of Amida Care, and, at the time of writing, their leaders comprised Amida Care's board.

Amida Care has an extensive network of primary care partners that bring specific expertise in the care of the chronically ill, whose diagnoses are often complicated by addiction, mental illness, and homelessness. Each primary care organization provided the following core services in ACCESS NY: HIV primary care, nursing medication management, medical social work, case management, outpatient mental health and adult day health care, health education, individual advocacy, benefit/entitlement assistance, escorts for medical care, assistance with finding and maintaining housing, and directly observed therapy that assisted clients in adhering to treatment.

1. *New York City AIDS Fund of the New York Community Trust (the Trust):* The Trust was the lead organization in ACCESS NY. It has extensive experience working with private funders, government officials, AIDS service representatives, and PLWH to review the status of the epidemic and make decisions about how private dollars can best be used to help PLWH. The Trust provided ongoing management and oversight of the project and had worked previously with Amida Care and PCDC in successful collaborations.

2. *Amida Care:* Amida Care is a Medicaid Special Needs Plan specially designed for PLWH. Its mission is to provide comprehensive care and coordinated services that facilitate improved health outcomes for its more than 5,600 members in NYC. The agency works with its members and providers to improve access to care, acting as the bridge between members and primary care providers. Amida Care has a history of successfully coordinating medical care and nonmedical needs such as the legal, housing, and case manage-

ment issues that many clients face. As part of ACCESS NY, Amida Care's role included identifying clients, referring them to primary care providers of their choosing, and providing them with the support to be retained in care. All CHOWs were based at Amida Care.

3. *Primary Care Development Corporation (PCDC)*: PCDC is a nonprofit organization dedicated to ensuring timely and effective access to primary care. Its mission is to invest in primary care facilities, improve service delivery, and lead policy initiatives. PCDC led the Learning Collaborative portion of the ACCESS NY project for the seven partner primary care provider organizations. In doing so, PCDC provided them with technical assistance to maximize clients' access to HIV medical care and to improve clinic and provider performance so as to facilitate clients' retention in care.

4. *Harlem United*: Harlem United is a Federally Qualified Health Center with medical and social support services for PLWH. Its clients face many barriers related to homelessness, addiction, mental illness, poverty, racial minority status, sexual orientation, and gender identity. Harlem United seeks to provide wraparound services in one location. Housing services include scattered site, transitional, and specialized women's housing. Additional supportive services include on-site psychiatry, dental care, mobile mental health counseling, crisis interventions, and food and nutrition services. Harlem United is an owner site of Amida Care, and a large percentage of its clients were Amida Care members. For ACCESS NY clients, Harlem United provided primary care.

5. *Housing Works*: Housing Works is a community-based organization dedicated to addressing the dual crises of AIDS and homelessness through advocacy and the provision of medical and social services, including entrepreneurial businesses. Specifically, its services include gynecology, chemical dependency services, a dental clinic, food and nutrition support, and extensive supportive housing. Housing Works has an access-to-care program that includes the Mobile Engagement Team, a mobile medical van, and other services for homeless people on the street. Housing Works is an owner site of Amida Care, and a large percentage of its clients were Amida Care members. As part of ACCESS NY, Housing Works provided care to ACCESS NY clients. Housing Works also had an on-site case manager who exclusively worked with Amida Care members.

6. *Help PSI / Project Samaritan*: Help PSI / Project Samaritan is a community-based organization that works to address HIV and substance use in the Bronx, Brooklyn, and Queens. Its services include a residential health care facility with a combined drug treatment program (66 beds), therapeutic community,

and a nursing home. The organization is an owner site of Amida Care, and a large percentage of its clients were Amida Care members. As part of ACCESS NY, Help PSI / Project Samaritan participated in the Learning Community and provided medical care to ACCESS NY clients.

7. *St. Mary's Episcopal Center:* St. Mary's Episcopal Center is a community-based organization focused on the long-term needs of individuals living with HIV. It is located in Central Harlem and provides a variety of services, including medical care, social services, and therapeutic recreation. The center also provides substance use counseling. St. Mary's is an owner of Amida Care, and a large percentage of its clients were also Amida Care members.

8. *Village Care of New York:* Village Care of New York is a long-term care facility serving seniors and individuals affected by HIV and AIDS who need continuing care or rehabilitation services. It has a skilled nursing facility (206 beds) with significant behavioral health and substance use interventions. Specific services provided include dental and gynecological care, food and nutrition services, specialized treatment adherence services, certified home health agency nursing, therapies, and mental health interventions in the home. Village Care is an owner site of Amida Care, and a large percentage of its clients were Amida Care members. ACCESS NY clients were frequently referred here for HIV treatment.

9. *Callen-Lorde*: Callen-Lorde is a health care provider for NYC's lesbian, gay, bisexual, and transgender (LGBT) community across all income levels. Its services include mental health services, dental services, HIV/AIDS facility-based care, and HIV testing. Callen-Lorde is a Federally Qualified Health Center that provides comprehensive, high-quality, and culturally sensitive medical care to meet the needs of the LGBT population. As part of the ACCESS NY network, Callen-Lorde provided LGBT-friendly medical care. A majority of its clients were Amida Care members. Callen-Lorde also had an on-site case manager who exclusively worked with Amida Care members.

10. *Acacia Network*: Acacia Network is a community-based organization that focuses on the needs of the Latino population by providing access to health services, housing, and economic opportunities. Services include health services, long-term care services, housing, case management, day programs, and vocational services. Acacia Network provided treatment and services for ACCESS NY clients.

Tables 7 and 8 summarize the characteristics of some of the New York City PC network sites and the services available to clients.

Table 7 Positive Charge (ACCESS NY) network partners, New York City

Organization	Legal fiscal designation	Type of health service agency*	Annual HIV operation budget	Number of PLWH served, 2010	Number of paid employees, 2010	Number of volunteers, 2010
Amida Care	Private, nonprofit	Medicaid Managed Care	~$30,270,000	1,200	68	0
Primary Care Development Corporation	Private, nonprofit	Performance improvement consultancy	~$800,000	n/a	30	n.d.
HELP PSI/Project Samaritan	Private, nonprofit	FQHC; FQMHC	n.d.	n.d.	n.d.	n.d.
Callen-Lorde	Private, nonprofit	FQHC	~$4,000,000	2,977	175	0

Note: Data were not available for the Trust, Harlem United, Housing Works, St. Mary's, Village Care, or the Acacia Network. n/a = not applicable; n.d. = no data available.

*FQHC = Federally Qualified Health Center; FQMHC = Federally Qualified Mental Health Center.

Table 8 Services offered to PLWH by ACCESS NY partner organizations, New York City

Organization	STI/HIV counseling and testing	HIV primary care	HIV case management	HIV outreach and linkage to care	HIV peer support	Other health services	Counseling services	HIV education and prevention services	Assistance with entitlement services	Support services*
Amida Care				×	×					
HELP PSI/Project Samaritan	×	×	×	×	×	×	×	×	×	H, T, N, S, ID
Callen-Lorde	×	×	×	×		×	×	×		

Note: PCDC is not a direct service provider (it is an advisor and leads the Access NY Learning Collaborative) and therefore is not included in the table. Data were not available for the Trust, Harlem United, Housing Works, St. Mary's, Village Care, or the Acacia Network.

*H = housing; ID = ID cards; N = nutritional support or food; S = substance use treatment; T = transportation.

The New York City AIDS Fund in the New York Community Trust

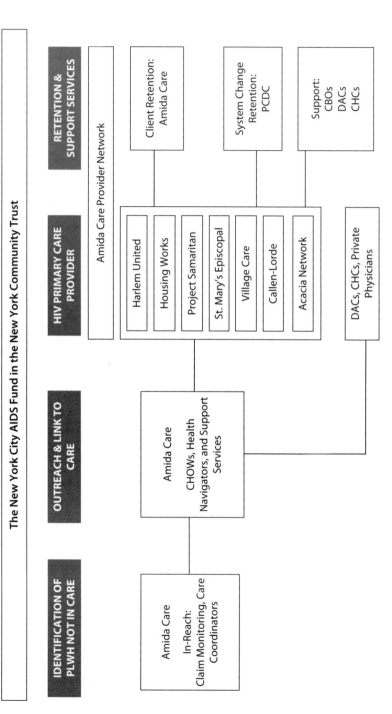

Figure 6. New York City Positive Charge network graphic

New York City Positive Charge Network
Network Graphic

Figure 6 depicts the ACCESS NY network. As represented by the long box at the top of the figure, the Trust played a key leadership role in overseeing implementation of the ACCESS NY program. The gray boxes indicate various steps or functions along the linkage-to-care continuum: identification of out-of-care PLWH through in-reach, outreach and linkage to services, provision of HIV primary care, and provision of support services. Organizations that fulfilled a particular function are listed below each gray box. Major organizations that were part of the ACCESS NY network are listed in boxes; other Amida Care organizations that were critical to the success of the project but were not ACCESS NY network members are grouped together in a larger box as "Amida Care Provider Network." Lines connecting boxes represent clients being referred from one collaborating organization to another for services along the linkage-to-care continuum.

The first column of the figure shows that Amida Care identified out-of-care PLWH primarily through its extensive roster of existing clients (in-reach). As an insurance provider, Amida Care has an electronic record of individuals who have not had a primary care visit claim in the past six months. As shown in the second column, individuals who were flagged in the Amida Care system were then referred to care coordinators who worked with CHOWs, health navigators, and other support service staff members to link PLWH back into care. If the individual had short-term, less intensive needs, they worked with a CHOW to link back into care. If the individual was identified as requiring more intensive linkage assistance (e.g., those with substance use, homelessness, or mental health issues), then they worked with a long-term care team to link back into care.

The program's key primary provider partners, who also participated in the Learning Collaborative (described below), were Harlem United, Housing Works, Project Samaritan, St. Mary's Episcopal, Village Care, Callen-Lorde, and Acacia Network. ACCESS NY also worked with other designated AIDS centers (DACs), community health centers (CHCs), and private doctors to link clients to a primary care provider. Decisions of where to link clients for HIV care were driven primarily by the preference of the participant and took into consideration clients' needs such as location and language services.

ACCESS NY also linked clients to a full range of support services, including housing, substance use, and mental health services, case management, and support groups. ACCESS NY also provided retention and support services: Amida Care worked to retain clients in care through long-term engagement. PCDC led the Learning Collaborative initiative by offering collaborative Learning Sessions to improve retention at the systems level. ACCESS NY collaborated with local community-based organizations (CBOs), DACs, and CHCs to provide additional support services to clients.

Internal Structural Changes

Respondents lauded the impact of ACCESS NY on their respective organizations. One respondent noted: "So what has come out of our participation in ACCESS NY is actually, like, huge; it's a whole new department" (Org. A). Following the inception of the program, the Retention and Care department at Org. A grew from a single-person operation to more than twenty personnel. This growth was accomplished with the help of additional grants. As a result of ACCESS NY and the needs identified through the program, five new non-PC programs were added under the new Retention and Care Unit. These included a program for individuals recently released from prison, in-house behavioral health services, and a staff member dedicated to housing. This organization also applied for a grant to support a women's health program for preventive care, such as mammograms and Pap smears. Org. A also planned to further leverage ACCESS NY to hire additional personnel through grant applications. In addition, the program helped to foster cross-departmental collaboration. A respondent noted that there had been a "cultural shift," in which different departments within the agencies and staff members of varying capacities were sharing information and resources to link potential clients into care. Org. A introduced a new "cluster" seating arrangement to further facilitate staff collaboration, where health navigators, nurses, case managers, and CHOWs all sat together and held case conferences each morning to discuss ongoing client issues. A respondent noted that they were constantly monitoring and reevaluating the processes in place to make them more efficient and streamlined: "We find that we're constantly re-tweaking to streamline it and to make it, for a lack of a better word, easier. So it's been a very interesting first for me, a year and a half just seeing these strategies re-tweaked and re-tooled and we keep forging on" (Org. A).

At Org. B and Org. C, respondents noted that ACCESS NY allowed the organizations to further leverage and strengthen the connections they already had with many shelters and community-based organizations. Through PCDC's Learning Collaborative, the program helped the organizations to introduce structural changes such as staffing changes, structural changes to waiting rooms, and staggered staff schedules: "They [PCDC] made sure that these clients were able to have access to our providers during given times or given schedules. They even arranged for transportation. ACCESS NY actually helped us develop some of the systems to become more patient-centered" (Org. B). Another change was an increased use of information technology:

> We had recently implemented an electronic medical record at the time we started with the ACCESS project, so it was very timely, because it helped us not only learn what we can get from the electronic medical record but to put the systems in place to help us utilize it a little bit more efficiently. They [PCDC] were very helpful and instrumental in helping us draft and test certain strategies to see what worked, what didn't, and what we eventually wound up with. —Org. B

The program also helped Org B. become more client-centered and facilitated its accreditation by the National Committee for Quality Assurance to become a Level 3 Patient-Centered Medical Home.

Identification of Clients

Org. A initially identified out-of-care PLWH through claims data. The organization kept track of those who had not had a claim for a doctor's visit within the past six months (seven months with one-month billing delay). As the program grew and became more established following its inception more than a decade earlier, providers and other departments in Org. A also referred potential clients identified as being out of care. These individuals were referred to the health navigators or CHOWs, who then made outreach calls to find potential clients, helped schedule first appointments, and sent transportation assistance (in the form of Metrocards), if necessary. These less intensive efforts were labeled Level-1 outreach. Potential clients identified as being out of care but needing more intensive assistance required Level-2 outreach. With Level-2 outreach, health navigators went out into the community to find clients who could not be reached over the phone and offered some field-based services, such as assessments and assistance with entitlements, medical appointments, and behavioral health appointments. These Level-2 efforts included short- and long-term case management tailored to the potential client's particular needs. Partner sites used a similar procedure to identify clients lost to care. They reviewed electronic medical records and patient management systems to identify these individuals.

Outreach and Linkage to Care

Respondents noted that before ACCESS NY, only minimal efforts were made to identify clients who were out of HIV care and link them back into care. There were no formal processes in place. Respondents mentioned that before ACCESS NY, they did not have the capacity to do more than simply enroll clients who did not have a doctor into Amida Care by making a referral to one of the primary care providers in its provider network. In fact, a respondent noted a stark contrast in protocol for how Amida Care worked with out-of-care clients before and after ACCESS NY:

> What we were doing back then is we would call people to say, "You need to go to the doctor," and if they didn't go to the doctor, then they would actually get disenrolled in the plan. And so we wouldn't follow them anymore. We wouldn't even know about them anymore. They were just gone . . . So it was really the opposite of what we're doing now. —Org. A

The intensive identification, outreach, linkage, and retention efforts for out-of-care clients of ACCESS NY were noted as being largely absent before the program began.

At Org. A, every month, each navigator was assigned ten referrals of individuals identified as out of care, in addition to the other clients with whom the navigator had been working for longer than a month. Each navigator had a caseload of about thirty clients, with each client at different stages of the linkage process. The navigator worked to help the referred individuals by identifying their needs and preferences and then tailored his or her recommendations or approach. Health navigators noted that their outreach and linkage efforts were not just about linking clients to medical care but also about helping to foster a sense of independence. One navigator noted: "I think it's really important that they're treated [by a provider] the same [way] without their advocate standing there and being in the shadows" (Org. A).

At the time of data collection, there were five CHOWs and seven health navigators, who were supervised by two managers. Both CHOWs and health navigators worked closely in a supportive environment, with each staff member focusing their attention on particular geographic regions or sites. Weekly meetings were also held to further ease collaboration. Staff members discussed their difficult cases so as to receive suggestions and tips and to learn about one another's areas of expertise (e.g., housing).

Org. A also introduced a new outreach strategy to seek potential clients who were identified as out of care and were admitted to a hospital. When a potential client was in the hospital, an on-call navigator was dispatched to speak with the individual about connecting into care. The health navigator would continue to help the client navigate health care systems after discharge from the hospital. The care coordination units or hospital made follow-up appointments for the client. The navigator escorted the client to the next primary care provider appointment.

All respondents agreed that the outreach and linkage process was intensive and often went beyond the first appointment with a primary care provider. As one health navigator noted: "Talking about getting to the bulb of an onion ... it's so layered and it's so complex, and that's life and that's people" (Org. A). Linkage went beyond medical care, to helping clients with other competing needs such as housing, mental health care, or substance use services. Case managers, primary care providers, and health navigators all worked together, sharing resources and client information. While respondents explained that it was extraordinarily difficult to link and engage with clients, they also mentioned that the challenge "means that we're not just cherry-picking. We really are looking for the hardest people to find ... 'If this wasn't a hard case, it would have never ended up on your desk. If we were getting the easy people, they don't need it'" (Org. A).

Org. B conducted outreach to local social service organizations such as shelters to build working relationships. Once these were established, Org. B would refer clients needing those services and receive referrals for clients needing HIV or mental health care. A respondent described this process:

> They [project staff] really actively went out and introduced themselves to new clients, new contacts, went into different hospitals, into newer community-based organizations that may have developed, the shelter systems ... they became the account manager for, say, [Shelter A] for clients that newly come in that need a medical and mental health evaluation in order to be placed appropriately for housing. —Org. B

Facilitators of PC Implementation

Respondents discussed the factors that facilitated implementation of AC-CESS NY. These factors included the Learning Sessions led by PCDC, collaboration across organizations, and support and buy-in from leadership and staff.

Learning Sessions

These sessions, held through the Learning Collaborative, were noted by many respondents as a factor that made ACCESS NY a success. As one interviewee noted, the sessions brought together different sets of staff, such as "nursing, medical providers, the front desk administrative staff. And then we actually had a frontline team member, so we had someone who worked on the front desk, one of the medical assistants" (Org. C), and taught them to work more effectively. PCDC helped organizations to streamline their work processes and created space to plan for rolling out these changes. An administrative staff member described new ways of evaluating and implementing changes in their project: "We learned new things every time we went [to the sessions]," particularly related to reviewing "where we are with some of the metrics, giving us insight into how we can finagle or change or maybe modify" (Org. B). Respondents noted that the Learning Sessions were an opportunity to learn not only from PCDC but also from other partner organizations that shared similar challenges "to hear how other places were approaching the very same issues you were, because you learned something they were doing that you could adopt or take" (Org. C).

Collaboration

Respondents explained that peer support among health navigators and CHOWs was constructive in helping link clients to care. Navigators would work together if potential clients were facing particular issues, such as domestic violence or substance use.

Org. A navigators worked with other departments within the agency and with other partner organizations. Different staff members worked together in identification, outreach, and linkage of a client into care, complementing one another's strengths and weaknesses. For example, a respondent stated that a CHOW with weaker administrative or office skills would be tapped to go out into the community to reach out to potential clients.

Connections among the organizations led to a helpful information exchange, as described by one respondent: "When you're able to call and ask for a specific person, you're able to get information that you need, and that makes it a lot easier" (Org. A). Organizations learned from one another's current practices: "[Org. D] came over to look at some of the systems that we have put in place . . . and we met and we went over certain things. Same thing with Org. E and Org C. We had Org C. come into some of our sites and talk about transgender" (Org. B).

It was also helpful for ACCESS NY organizations to hear about the challenges and strategies of other grantees in the PC network; these discussions helped to manage expectations and shed light on how different sites were handling their own struggles "so they understand that it's a hard-to-engage population sometimes. It may take longer than 30 days to get them [clients] into care" (Org. A).

Support from leadership and funders

An administrative staff member emphasized that having the complete support of management was the biggest facilitator in the success of the program. Management readily provided the funding, resources, and guidance. Without this, the program would probably have stalled and collapsed, according to the respondent. Support from and open discussions with the funder, AIDS United, were also cited as a facilitator.

Staff buy-in/awareness

Buy-in, at both service delivery and leadership levels, was paramount in ACCESS NY's success. Initially, staff were reluctant to buy into the process, but through weekly meetings and status updates, efforts were made to involve staff in implementing the ACCESS NY program and to incorporate their feedback. As the systems began to show improvement and staff understood the need for the changes, there was better buy-in. It was also helpful for ACCESS NY to hear about the challenges and strategies of other grantees in the PC network.

Unmet Client Needs and Barriers to PC Implementation

Respondents reported that the primary barriers and challenges to implementation of ACCESS NY were health information technology, collaborating with partner organizations, appropriateness of standard operating procedures, and competing client needs.

Health information technology

Respondents noted their frustrations with being unable to capture all the efforts made by staff to engage with clients and link them to care as a result of flaws in the data management system. Org. A's system was not built to handle the large amounts of data that were generated by the project: "I don't think that anyone really recognized how quickly we would grow and what it would mean . . . so there's data that we may not necessarily have a good way of getting" (Org. A). The system was also "homegrown" and was not necessarily built to develop progress reports: "We have a homegrown database that was made for us and not necessarily to report out and certainly not to report out the kind of data that we are currently reporting out" (Org. A). As a result of these issues, it took some time for the organizations to establish a protocol to provide monitoring and evaluation reports for program management and the data reports required by all PC sites. Respondents also noted that staff had some difficulty becoming oriented to the new electronic medical record.

Data were also an issue for partner organizations participating in the Learning Collaborative with PCDC. PCDC asked the organizations to monitor seven measures, such as cycle time and time to third-next available appointment, and to track system-level changes at each partner organization. A respondent noted that staff had trouble understanding what the various constructs meant and how they were calculated. It was only after extensive efforts were made to draw links between the various measures and how they benefited clients' care experience that staff became more enthusiastic and committed to collecting data. A respondent commented that "once some of the systems actually started to show improvement and people had a better understanding of why we were badgering them about cycle time, or measuring their cycle time from in and out, to understand how it relates to capacity and then how the capacity relates to having better access, there was a better buy-in" (Org. F).

Collaboration with partner organizations

Respondents noted that it was sometimes challenging to work with partner organizations that were unaware of who the CHOWs or health navigators were. As a result, staff at these organizations were reluctant to share client information or resources. Respondents felt that this was probably due to the high turnover in some organizations:

So, I do feel like we're part of the network, but I feel like sometimes when that key person is not there, the access doesn't flow as freely as it should. And I think it should be across the board, everybody knows that this is the managed care program. They call, and they give you the specifics. You are able to speak with them. So, I don't know how that would look. Maybe . . . monthly education to the organization about our partnership and our network. —Org. A

Standard operating procedures

Organizations reported that, at times, the standardized definitions in the project acted as a barrier. For example, "linkage to care" was defined as a visit with an HIV medical care provider within thirty days of enrollment. Organizations found that achieving this goal was difficult, and being measured against such a challenging target became demoralizing for staff. In another example, staff explained that their interaction with clients often went beyond the first appointment or linkage of a client to care. A respondent said: "We don't feel so comfortable with closing the case out . . . because I feel, and I think we all feel, that they're just getting started. They're on the road to being engaged" (Org. A). For the respondents, it was not enough just to get a client to the first appointment, given that these individuals often grappled with other problems such as homelessness, poverty, or substance use.

A health navigator noted that "we are working with people that have a thousand and one different other things going on. So, I think if I was able to, I would extend that [thirty-day period]. It shouldn't be a failure because you're not able to get them in within that timeframe" (Org. A). Given these issues, outreach and linkage staff had to develop trust with clients and help tackle the other barriers.

Respondents also noted that strictly adhering to the enrollment criteria— to include only those who were deemed to be out of care for six months—was morally difficult:

And so that is someone who we don't want to wait until they're out of care for six months. We want to get them enrolled in services now. And we've just started doing that because I couldn't in good faith say, "No. Sorry. We have to wait three more months until that person is really lost before we can get them." —Org. A

Client needs and attitudes

Respondents overwhelmingly reported that clients often faced a barrage of issues that acted as barriers to engagement in care, and staff members had to make intense efforts to identify, reach out to, and link someone with their first medical appointment. As one respondent explained: "We've had people say, 'I don't want to go to the doctor. I want to sit in my apartment and smoke crack until I die.' And I'm not exaggerating, people have said that or, like, 'Who cares about me?'" (Org. A). Competing client needs were also frequently mentioned:

> There's motivated patients, and then there are patients who are dealing with many other things, like not having a place to live, not having food, not having a job, and that interferes with their ability to make their health care a priority when they're dealing with such basic needs. —Org. C

One particular need was overwhelmingly cited as unmet: housing. A respondent estimated that more than 60% of clients needed housing assistance. While many services and programs are offered in New York City, respondents noted that clients were often unaware of them. These services and programs are difficult to navigate and access, with some only accessible through public assistance. Care for hepatitis C co-infections was also cited as an unmet need among clients.

Overarching Conclusions

Following implementation of ACCESS NY, there was a new focus on retaining clients in HIV primary care. Org. A had a department focused on retention and care that grew significantly, as well as several new projects based on this new expertise. Collaboration increased within the lead agency and across the partner agencies, particularly through the PCDC Learning Collaborative. Organizations shared their experiences and challenges and worked to modify processes as their clinics sought to boost access for clients served by ACCESS NY. New techniques for identification and linkage were also explored, such as working with clients soon to be discharged from the hospital.

A key challenge in implementing the project was that clients were difficult to find, often did not want to seek care, and faced many competing barriers, including housing. Housing was particularly difficult to address due to the extremely high housing costs in NYC. Some of the implementation procedures were challenging for staff, such as the thirty-day limit for linking clients to care. Other challenges for project staff were related to data management tools and timely, complete reporting. It was also difficult to train staff in understanding and collecting data. Collaboration posed a challenge, too, particularly in establishing partners' understanding of the roles of the community health outreach workers.

Despite the problems and challenges, respondents were enthusiastic and believed in the program. Health navigators and CHOWs felt they had a positive influence on clients' lives. One respondent summarized their experience with the project in this way:

> I really believe in this program . . . And members really appreciate it, clients really appreciate it. You know, it's someone from your health plan who they would never . . . suspect that they would care, coming out and saying, look we care about you . . . Sometimes health care becomes the last thing you think about . . . I think this is about helping people give people tools to help. —Org. A

San Francisco / Bay Area

Background

California had 49,473 total cumulative HIV cases from April 2006 to December 31, 2013, when the disease was first reported by name. California also had 168,602 total cumulative AIDS cases from the beginning of the epidemic to December 31, 2013 (California Department of Public Health [CDPH] 2013). The state was second only to New York State in the number of living individuals diagnosed with HIV (at any stage of disease) as of the end of 2010 (Centers for Disease Control and Prevention 2011a). Men faced the largest HIV and AIDS burden in California, accounting for 89.4% of cumulative cases as of December 31, 2013. HIV and AIDS are distributed across racial groups, with 50.6% of HIV or AIDS cases among Whites, 27.0% among Hispanics, and 17.8% among Black/African Americans. Individuals over 30 years of age accounted for the majority of infections, with 39.6% of infections occurring among the 30 to 39 age group, 27.2% among the 40 to 49 age group, and 13.0% among persons over the age of 49. The majority of infections (66.6%) were believed to be transmitted by unprotected intercourse among men who have sex with men (MSM) (CDPH 2013).

San Francisco is the county with the second-largest number of people living with HIV and AIDS (5,813 and 9,623, respectively, in 2013) in California (CDPH 2013). The epidemiologic profile of people living with HIV and AIDS in San Francisco is similar to that for the rest of California. The greatest burden of disease is carried by men (92%), and the most common means of exposure is MSM (73%). The number of newly diagnosed HIV cases has steadily decreased over time, from 513 in 2008, to 463 in 2009, 434 in 2010, and 409 in 2011. The number of AIDS diagnoses per year has also fallen annually since 1993 (San Francisco Department of Public Health [SFDPH] 2012).

Community viral load (CVL) is the average of the most recent viral loads of all people living with HIV (PLWH) in a particular geographic location (e.g., the Castro neighborhood) or of a group of people who share a certain characteristic (e.g., MSM). A 2010 study of San Francisco found that the mean CVL for Black/African Americans, Latinos, women, transgender individuals, people who inject drugs (PWID), and MSM-PWID were higher than the mean CVL for the San Francisco PLWH population as a whole. Individuals who were in care and receiving treatment had a lower mean CVL than the population of PLWH living in San Francisco overall. When CVL was examined by location, researchers found that homeless individuals had the highest CVL, followed by individuals who lived in southeast Bayview, a lower-income area with a primarily Black/African American population (Das et al. 2010).

California received $433,469,436 in HIV and AIDS federal grant funding in FY 2012. The state received $71,758,702 from the Centers for Disease Control and Prevention and $300,012,288 in Ryan White HIV/AIDS Program funding. Other major federal funds were from the Housing Opportunities for Persons with AIDS ($39,343,180), Substance Abuse and Mental Health Services Administration ($21,545,633), and Office of Minority Health ($809,633) (Kaiser Family Foundation 2012). California had 41,179 individuals enrolled in the AIDS Drug Assistance Program in FY 2010 and spent more than any other state on medications for HIV ($40,300,136) during FY 2011 (NASTAD 2012).

Program Overview

The Positive Charge (PC) project implemented in the Bay Area/San Francisco was the Bay Area Network for Positive Health (BANPH). BANPH worked with highly underserved populations, including PLWH who were in poverty, transitioning out of jail or prison, substance users, transgender individuals, and people of color. The intervention coordinated the efforts of multiple agencies to locate individuals who were out of care, to strengthen peer and social networks, and to reduce provider-based barriers.

The project was structured into a formal network of community based organizations (CBOs) and clinical partners and was coordinated by a team at the Health Equity Institute of San Francisco State University (HEI). The BANPH lead team consisted of a network coordinator, an evaluation coordinator, an outreach coordinator, an administrative and data management assistant, and a linkage specialist. The BANPH network consisted of partners who were or were not receiving funds. Only subgrantees were approached for the purposes of this analysis.

Positive Charge Partner Organizations

At the time this case study was completed, BANPH was a consortium comprising nine organizations and one program working together to link PLWH into care. The network included two health departments, four community-based social service organizations, one health center, one program, and one academic institution, as described below.

1. *Health Equity Institute for Research, Policy, and Practice (HEI):* Located at San Francisco State University, HEI aims to improve health and eliminate health disparities through research, training, community outreach, technical assistance, and dissemination. It has a focus on social justice and equity. HEI was the lead agency in BANPH. It also conducted outreach and received referrals from organizations outside BANPH.

2. *Alameda County Public Health Department (ACPHD):* The mission of ACPHD is to work with the community to ensure optimal health and well-being. The health department serves three core functions: assessment, including ongoing collection, analysis, and sharing of information about health risks and health resources; policy development driven by assessment; and assurance focused on maintaining the capacity of the department to respond to critical situations. The Office of AIDS Administration, which is embedded within the ACPHD, seeks to reduce HIV infections, increase awareness of HIV serostatus, and provide timely linkage to care for PLWH. As part of the PC program, ACPHD's role was to conduct outreach and linkage-to-care activities for clients referred by medical providers. A disease intervention specialist was assigned to ACPHD to help with these activities.

3. *Centerforce:* Centerforce is a nonprofit community-based organization that seeks to support, educate, and advocate for individuals, families, and communities affected by incarceration. The organization develops, implements, and evaluates programs that foster transformative experiences during incarceration, promotes ties between incarcerated individuals and their families, assists individuals with accessing services before and during reentry, provides support to individuals affected by incarceration, and provides education about health concerns that disproportionately affect incarcerated populations.

Within the BANPH network, Centerforce worked with incarcerated individuals living with HIV who were being released from San Quentin State Prison to provide referral and linkage-to-care support.

4. *Forensic AIDS Project (FAP):* FAP is a program of Jail Health Services that operates in the San Francisco City and County jails. Run by the San Francisco Department of Public Health, the program is designed for incarcerated individuals who are living with HIV or at risk for acquiring HIV. Interventions include HIV testing, linkage to and engagement in care, jail-based drug treatment, and outreach to substance users housed in intake housing units. As part of the PC project, FAP conducted in-reach within the San Francisco county jail to link inmates to HIV services while incarcerated and after reentry into the community.

5. *Mission Neighborhood Health Center (MNHC):* MNHC is a 39-year-old community-based health center within the Mission community of San Francisco. The health center provides comprehensive primary health care services, gynecological and prenatal care, and pediatric services. It has four locations, including the Excelsior Clinic, which provides adult and youth preventive medicine services such as physical exams, cancer screening, vaccinations, and family planning. MNHC's Clinica Esperanza provides HIV prevention and treatment services to meet the needs of the Latino community. The clinic currently provides medical services, case management, health education, nutritional counseling, medication adherence services, and peer advocacy to more than 400 clients living with HIV. As part of the PC program, MNHC enrolled eligible individuals who were receiving its services and conducted in-reach to existing out-of-care clients to ensure adequate HIV care and retention in care.

6. *San Francisco AIDS Foundation (SFAF):* SFAF was founded in 1982 with a mission to reduce new HIV infections in San Francisco. The organization has three goals: to reduce new HIV infections in San Francisco by 50%, to ensure that all San Franciscans know their current HIV status, and to ensure access to proper care for all San Franciscans living with HIV. SFAF aims to meet these goals through education, advocacy, and direct services. Its programs include support groups, case management, peer advocacy, HIV testing, needle exchange, substance use and mental health education and services, advocacy, and education. During the PC project, SFAF identified PWID clients through extensive street-based outreach and linked them to care, as well as conducting in-reach to clients who accessed syringe exchange services.

7. *San Francisco Department of Public Health (SFDPH):* The mission of SFDPH is to protect and promote the health of all persons living in San Francisco. The department has two primary divisions: the Community Health Network and Population, Health, and Prevention. The department's programs include HIV testing, linkage to care, prevention services, policy and advocacy, implementation and evaluation research, and substance use research. As part of BANPH, SFDPH used department surveillance data on HIV cases and data from HIV reporting lab results to provide information on retention in care of linked clients.

8. *Street Level Health Project (SLHP):* SLHP is a community-based organization that aims to improve the health and well-being of underserved urban immigrants in the Bay Area. The SLHP community center provides health care and social services, including a health screening clinic, health navigators, and temporary assistance for those with basic needs such as food and clothing. In addition, SLHP engages in advocacy and coalition building. The health screening drop-in clinic provides basic diagnostic and treatment services; referrals to primary, specialty, and urgent care; mental health services; and case management. Clinic services are offered in Spanish, English, Mongolian, Man, Nepali, Chinese, and Vietnamese to meet the diverse language needs of their clients. As part of BANPH, SLHP conducted extensive street outreach to Latino day laborers in Oakland and enrolled its existing clients into the PC project to access free medical care, meals, and groups.

9. *Women Organized to Respond to Life Threatening Diseases (WORLD):* WORLD was founded in 1991 to provide services to women living with and affected by HIV. With a focus on women and families, WORLD provides a range of services, including peer advocacy, outreach, a speakers bureau, client and community retreats, and the Positive Women's Network, a network of women that aims to support women living with HIV in leadership roles and to shape federal policy. During the PC program, WORLD followed up with women referred to its services from outside medical providers and other service providers.

Tables 9 and 10 summarize the characteristics of partner organizations in BANPH and the services they offered to clients.

San Francisco / Bay Area Positive Charge Network
Network Graphic

Figure 7 depicts the BANPH network. As represented by the long box at the top of the figure, HEI played a key leadership role in overseeing implementation

Table 9 Positive Charge (BANPH) network partners, San Francisco/Bay Area

Organization	Legal fiscal designation	Type of health service agency	Annual HIV operation budget	PLWH served, 2010	Paid employees, 2010	Volunteers, 2010
HEI	Public	Academic institution	~$114,000	12	6	n/a
ACPHD	Public	Health department	n.d.	n.d.	n.d.	n/a
Centerforce	Private nonprofit	Social service organization	~$1.9 million (overall)*	n.d.	39*	25*
FAPt	Public	Program of the SFDPH	~$1 million	727	11	4
MNHC	Public	Community health center	~$11 million (overall)*	400	250	5*
SFAF	Private nonprofit	Social service organization	~$21 million*	n.d.	127*	9,467*
SFDPH	Public	Health department	n.d.	n.d.	n.d.	n/a
SLHP	Private nonprofit	Social service organization	$20,500	n.d.	7	1,560
WORLD	Private nonprofit	Social service organization	n.d.	300	13	2

Note: All organization names are given in full in the text. n/a = not applicable; n.d. = no data available.
*Information from form 990 (MNHC 2009; SFAF 2010; Centerforce 2011).

Table 10 Services offered to PLWH by BANPH network organizations

Organization	STI/HIV counseling and testing	HIV primary care	HIV case management	HIV outreach and linkage to care	HIV peer support	Other health services	Counseling services	HIV education and prevention services	Assistance with entitlement services	Support services*
HEI				✕			✕			
Centerforce			✕	✕	✕		✕			
FAP	✕	✕	✕	✕		✕	✕	✕	✕	H, T, N, S
MNHC	✕	✕	✕	✕	✕	✕	✕	✕		N, S
SLHP				✕	✕	✕	✕	✕		N

Note: Data were not available for ACPHD, SFAF, SFDPH, or WORLD; therefore, these organizations are not included in the table. All organization names are given in full in the text.

*H = housing; N = nutritional support or food; S = substance use treatment; T = transportation.

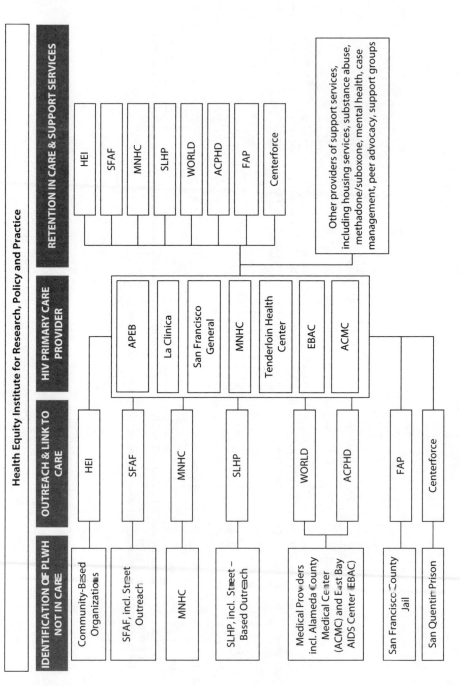

Figure 7. Bay Area Network for Positive Health network graphic

of the BANPH project. The gray boxes indicate various steps or functions along the linkage-to-care continuum: identification of PLWH who are out of care, outreach and linkage to care, provision of HIV primary care, and provision of support services. Organizations that fulfilled a particular function are listed below each gray box. Lines connecting boxes show organizations working together to refer patients from one organization to another for services along the linkage-to-care continuum.

The first two columns of the figure show that HEI, WORLD, ACPHD, FAP, and Centerforce worked with partners to identify and conduct outreach to seek individuals who were out of care. For example, HEI conducted outreach to and received referrals from CBOs that were not part of BANPH. SLHP and MNHC primarily enrolled clients who received health-related services at their facilities. SLHP also conducted extensive street-based outreach, as did SFAF. The second column lists the eight organizations that linked individuals into care as part of the BANPH project. BANPH partners simultaneously linked PLWH to HIV primary care services and to support services. BANPH linked clients to a range of HIV primary care providers throughout Oakland and San Francisco, including AIDS Project of East Bay (APEB), La Clinica, San Francisco General Health, MNHC, and Tenderloin Health Center, to name a few. Decisions about where to link clients for HIV care were driven primarily by clients' preference and considered needs such as location and language services. BANPH also linked clients to a full range of support services, including housing, substance use treatment, mental health services, case management, and support groups.

Network Sociogram

Figure 8 is a sociogram of the BANPH network in October 2011, during the PC project. The network has a density of 0.64, meaning that it includes 64% of all possible ties. The average degree, or average number of ties per organization, is 4.5. The network centralization was 33%, meaning that while some organizations reported more connections than others, no single organization was responsible for most or all of the connections between organizations.

We also assessed connectedness between BANPH partner agencies six months before the start of PC. Specifically, we asked organizations whether they had worked with any of the partner agencies in the six months prior to BANPH to link PLWH into care. As seen in figure 9, the pre-BANPH network was not nearly as connected: density is 0.25; average node degree is 1.8; and network centralization is 81%, meaning that one organization was responsible for most of the connections.

Following implementation of PC, then, network centralization decreased dramatically from 81% to 33%, meaning that partner organizations connected with other partners without the lead agency, HEI, acting as facilitator. Similarly, density increased from 0.25 to 0.64, meaning that the percentage of all

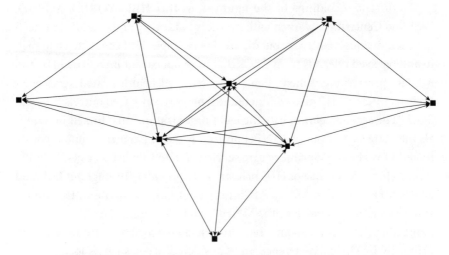

Figure 8. Bay Area Network for Positive Health network sociogram

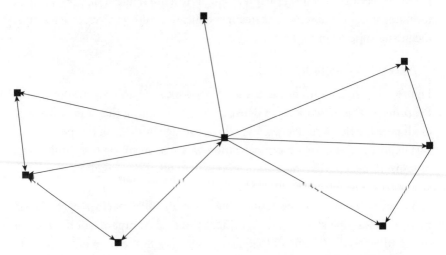

Figure 9. Bay Area organizational network sociogram six months before
Positive Charge

possible ties increased from 25% to 64%. Taken together, the changes in network centralization and density score across the BANPH network suggest tighter linkages and increased collaboration within the PC network.

Internal Structural Changes

Organizations reported a variety of internal structural changes resulting from the BANPH program. The most frequently reported structural change across all organizations was the addition of staff. As a result of BANPH, organizations were able to hire new staff to conduct linkage-to-care activities.

The BANPH organizations also reported a limited number of internal structural changes to their health care delivery systems. For example, Org. H incorporated information about HIV testing into its preventive health screener to promote dialogue with clients about HIV. Org. C, which provides services within jails, made changes to its intake system: the responsibility for client intake was transferred to the organization's linkage-to-care coordinator. As a result, Org. C was able to contact all individuals who were potentially eligible for BANPH. This change in responsibilities allowed Org. C to reach out to a population of PLWH it was not able to work with previously: individuals who had been incarcerated for less than 72 hours.

Identification of Clients

A variety of strategies to identify PLWH who were out of care were reported, including referrals, in-reach, and outreach.

Referrals

Most organizations relied on referrals to identify out-of-care PLWH. The BANPH network received referrals from HIV testing sites, HIV primary care providers, and social service organizations. A respondent at one organization described the process of disseminating information about the project to encourage referrals:

> We would go to all these agencies, just to let them know who BANPH was and what we do and what our goals were and to let them know that if they have clients that are HIV positive, and out of care, they can refer these clients to us. So I went to homeless shelters, churches, community centers. I've been to needle exchanges, day labor, soup kitchens, and HIV testing sites. So I've been really developing my relationship with all these different agencies—Mother Brown's

Place, where they had a Veterans' program. So if they had clients that are positive, they were referred to us. —Org. D

In-reach

Several organizations reported that they used in-reach as a strategy to identify PLWH in need of BANPH services. One in-reach method was the cre-
ation of a list of existing or former clients who were out of care or in need of
linkage-to-care services. This list of names and contact information became
a starting point for outreach efforts to find potential clients.

Outreach

Organizations employed a variety of outreach strategies to identify out-of-
care PLWH, including street-based, community-based, and network-based
outreach. Some organizations used outreach strategies to simultaneously
provide information and education, raise awareness about HIV and HIV
testing, and identify potential BANPH clients. Outreach activities included
presentations to community groups and street-based condom distribution as
a platform to spread the word about the BANPH program. Organizations also
engaged in traditional "pounding the pavement" outreach, as one interviewee
explained:

> I go out to the street in the mornings, Monday, Tuesday, Wednesday, and find
> the guys. He [another staff member from Org. H] kind of hooks on to when they
> are giving out the breakfast. [He] talks to them about HIV, about STDs . . . They
> give out information on services. I mostly talk about getting tested for HIV [and]
> using condoms. They can always call me or come here to find me. —Org H.

Lastly, one organization indicated that its peers used a network-based approach to identify individuals in need of care and treatment. This organization
had trained its peers to work within their social networks to provide information and education on HIV and to connect friends and family who were living
with HIV and were out of care back into HIV care and treatment.

Across the BANPH network, most organizations used a variety of strategies to identify out-of-care individuals, based on the idea that using multiple
strategies helped them to reach a diverse population that included the most
underserved. The organizations that relied primarily on outreach champi-
oned this method to reach those most difficult to find, but all recognized the
importance of working with clinics, prisons, jails, or health departments be-

cause these had access to contact information for out-of-care individuals who would benefit from services provided by BANPH. The BANPH organizations could then conduct recruitment through in-reach. Organizations that employed such strategies, in particular those that worked with incarcerated populations, explained the benefit and convenience of this strategy. As one respondent noted: "The need is there . . . I don't have to go recruit someone randomly or have networks out to try to find someone—the people are sitting right there in front of us" (Org. B).

Identification and initial contact usually did not happen simultaneously. Rather, organizations would have a name from in-reach or from a referral. Out-of-care individuals did not usually present themselves to the organization, and the organization was tasked with finding them. One respondent explained:

> And when I say out of care, I mean, haven't seen their doctor [in] more than six months to probably a year or two and no one knows how to find them . . . And BANPH gives me the opportunity to go out there and find these [individuals], make connection with these [individuals], link them back to care. —Org. I

Outreach and Linkage to Care

Linkage was seen as a multistage process that included steps such as making initial contact with the individual, building rapport, linking to social services, and finally, linking to HIV primary care. Organizations that worked with incarcerated populations stressed the importance of making initial contact with potential clients before their release. They found that when an initial introduction happened on the "inside," follow-up with clients on the "outside" was much more successful.

All BANPH organizations found that their initial contact with clients was critical for establishing trust and rapport. Some characteristics of initial contact that helped to build positive relationships were having in-person meetings and meeting at a location that was comfortable and convenient for the potential client:

> Just be willing to meet the clients, [somewhere] where they are happy. Because if you're telling them, oh, you have to meet me at this office . . . they don't want to come down there . . . Okay. I don't mind spending two or three dollars out of my own pocket to engage with you if you are willing to meet them where they're at . . . I think it's much better. If you're willing to take a little extra time,

to meet with the clients where they are at and make it a little bit more comfortable for them, that is something else. You'll be successful. —Org. C

Respondents described the importance of recognizing clients' priorities. They found it was often beneficial to identify and address clients' needs as a precursor to linkage to HIV care:

As we know from the purpose of linkages, that why we need linkage is that we know the [client's] priority is very rarely care. The priority is much more survival based, much more right now in the moment focused, [on] immediate needs. So my goal is never to change their minds about their priorities but to engage in more of a negotiation, so my priority is to engage them in care. I don't expect their priorities to change. I want to learn what their priorities are and I want to meet their needs. —Org. B

Across all organizations in the study, linking clients to support services was an important step in the linkage-to-care continuum because this step addressed the factors that kept individuals out of care. In addition, organizations reported that successful linkage to support services helped to build rapport and legitimacy with clients because it allowed the organization to demonstrate to clients that it could deliver services that met their perceived needs.

In discussing linkages to HIV primary care, three themes emerged: tailoring referrals to clients, attending appointments with clients, and following up with organizations after referrals had been made. Respondents discussed the importance of tailoring the HIV health care linkage to the needs and concerns of the client. As one interviewee explained:

As far as care or the linkage portion of it . . . we've had individuals who come in who don't want anything AIDS-related in the title. Like, they won't go to an agency that has AIDS in the title. "I don't want to go to an agency that's anywhere near, you know, Oakland, I don't want anybody to know" . . . a whole possible list of concerns that any particular individual may have as far as just linking them to care. So if it's just linking them directly into medical care after hearing what some of their concerns are, we are able to then say, well, okay, [name of health center] sounds like it'll be a good fit for you. Or [name of health center] may be a good fit for you." —Org. A

Across organizations, staff described the process of making appointments for BANPH clients and attending HIV primary care and treatment appointments with their clients. They attended these appointments both to provide emotional support and to help individuals navigate the HIV health care delivery system. After making appointments and referrals, following up with agencies where the referrals were made was important. As one respondent commented:

> So it is not hard for me to call somebody at [name of hospital] and say can so-and-so come to the appointment, did they make the appointment? Because they [the client] will come and say, oh yeah, I made the appointment, but I'll call . . . the clinic and just check in . . . we're all kind of connected. —Org. C

Respondents explained that linkage to care was a multistage process that went beyond simply referring someone to a primary care provider. For BANPH organizations, linkage to care included identifying and locating individuals who were out of care; building rapport and relationships with clients; identifying barriers to care and linkage to support services; making, attending, and following up on HIV medical appointments; and providing ongoing support.

Most organizations indicated that they had done HIV linkage-to-care work before the PC project. For these organizations (Org. A, Org. B, Org. C, Org. I), BANPH either was complementary to their ongoing work or provided funding to continue linkage-to-care work that had ceased. For example, Org. I had previously worked on a project to link women with high viral loads back into care. Org. B had a long history of providing linkage-to-care services through transitional case management, but due to changes in the way transitional case management was being implemented, the organization was no longer providing this service. Org. C was well versed in providing HIV prevention and care services to incarcerated adults and coordinated case management following release. In contrast, Org. H had expertise in linking clients to medical care and services but was new to working in the area of HIV care.

Facilitators of PC Implementation

Staff at the BANPH organizations discussed the factors that facilitated program implementation, factors that operated across the organizational, program, and individual levels. These included relationships with medical and support service organizations, strong collaboration within the BANPH network, incentives for clients, peers' sharing their own experiences with clients, and staff expertise.

Having strong relationships with social support and HIV service organizations emerged as an important element for program implementation. These relationships existed before BANPH and were with non-BANPH organizations, but they greatly facilitated implementation:

> One of the things that's really made things easier is to really know local resources. Not only know the local resources but have a connection with them so that when you call them when somebody is homeless, you can actually get somebody into care, that you can address those barriers. —Org. A

Organizations found that having strong relationships with non-BANPH agencies helped to ensure successful connections to either HIV care or support services. Strong relationships also allowed continued client follow-up after linkages had been made. Related to this theme was the importance of having a formal structure in place between organizations that allowed sharing of client-level information. Some organizations, such as health departments, came into BANPH with these systems already in place within existing organizational structures:

> One of the best things that has come to light for us is that once again we are the public health department so we have access to information without having to violate an individual's confidentiality or to have some type of MoU [memorandum of understanding] to access information. So for us, we can take a name and go through the state's HARS [Enhanced HIV/AIDS Reporting System] program and find out when an individual's last labs were done. We can also work with our vital records to see if an individual has passed away. We can also work with our STD/HIV surveillance unit to ID an individual, like where they live, through DMV [Department of Motor Vehicle] records, so we have potentially a number of avenues of whittling down the list. So I would suggest, or [make a] recommendation, if an agency has the opportunity to really partner with the public health department, and if there is specifically an AIDS office, an office of AIDS administration, it does really increase the avenues of information. —Org. A

In discussing organizational relationships *within* the BANPH network, respondents noted that their organization did not share client-level information within the network because MoUs or similar release-of-client-information systems were not in place. Some organizations saw this as a weakness of the network and as a barrier to efficient program implementation. For example, some agencies reported that they were potentially looking for and serving the same clients and had no means to verify whether or not this was the case. While some respondents felt that their organization worked "in a silo" and did not collaborate with other BANPH organizations, others indicated that BANPH provided structure at the organizational level, primarily by holding monthly meetings where BANPH partners could share information about their programs and services.

At the program level, organizations reported various strategies that helped them to link clients to care successfully. A common theme emerged around the importance of providing client incentives. The lead agency provided partner agencies with incentives to give to BANPH clients, including a $10 card for the supermarket, string backpack, stress ball, notebook, pen, and calendar. Some organizations included additional incentives such as transportation tokens and gift cards to Goodwill and fast-food restaurants. As one interviewee explained:

> I really thought incentives. Something nice, too, and . . . not just no gift card . . . Socks, lotion, body gel, ChapStick, stress ball, foot cream, body sprays . . . And what happens is some women really appreciate that. And they want to come back just because you was kind enough to do all this. —Org. I

In addition to tangible incentives such as gift cards and goods, organizations noted that providing clients with high-quality linkages to social services also served as a "hook" or an incentive.

The peer model emerged as a strategy that promoted successful implementation. Peers were lauded because of their ability to relate with clients, to provide firsthand experience and knowledge, and to provide leadership. As one respondent noted:

> The thing . . . we like about peers is that oftentimes the peers have gone through . . . a number of the presenting barriers. What better way to really work with somebody . . . to have someone say, I've been there . . . I know where you're coming from, but this is how we move your life forward. —Org. A

Another respondent expanded on this:

> [Our organization has] a peer navigator who already knows that HIV health care system . . . and is Spanish speaking and does get services in this county. There is less that he has to learn because he has already been through everything, he has been in the system for five years at least. So I think that has been

a big benefit for our organization. And he is an immigrant. I think that [having] someone from the community, having the popular opinion leader, is the key. That is the number one. —Org. H

At the individual level, respondents discussed the importance of the characteristics and expertise of linkage staff in facilitating program implementation, as well as the benefit of having staff who were tenacious and passionate about their work. In working with clients, the importance of having built rapport with them by being nonjudgmental, trustworthy, and reliable was mentioned. Finally, linkage-to-care staff were able to draw on their previous background and experience to inform the work that they did for BANPH. For example, respondents indicated that previous experience in fields such as public health investigation and nursing was beneficial to the program.

A respondent noted the importance of a program's past experience in working in linkage to care and in working with the population of focus:

So I think for us, [an advantage is] the fact that we already work with this population and we have the experience, so I think anyone that has never worked [in this area], like a brand new organization trying to do this work, I think the amount of time that it takes to build ... relationships with stakeholders, and figure out systems, is—I don't even think it could be done. —Org. C

In summary, at the program level, two overarching facilitating factors emerged: use of incentives and the peer model. At the individual level, organizations noted the characteristics and expertise of linkage staff that were necessary for successful program implementation, such as passion, tenacity, trustworthiness, reliability, and prior experience working with this population.

Unmet Client Needs and Barriers to PC Implementation

The primary barriers to program implementation, as reported by the BANPH organizations, included barriers at the systems level and barriers related to the client context.

System-level barriers

Respondents at the organizations that worked with incarcerated and formerly incarcerated populations spoke frequently about the challenges that accompanied working within the jail and prison systems. These challenges were particularly great for newly hired staff. It took time to learn the often

complex systems that govern jails and prisons. It was challenging to forge relationships with prison/jail staff who did not initially understand the benefit
of linkage to care. Lastly, organizations faced challenges in navigating the
prison systems. Tasks such as visiting clients were sometimes made difficult
by unanticipated events (e.g., lockdowns). One organization discussed its
struggle to establish a system to ensure that medical records were available
for incarcerated individuals for periods in and out of prison.

Client context

The context surrounding BANPH's clients also created challenges. BANPH
served highly vulnerable populations. Organizations communicated that
working to address the priorities of clients who had multiple unmet basic
needs was difficult. Also highlighted was that the clients they worked with
faced HIV-related stigma and were distrustful of medical systems. These factors were ongoing barriers to clients' receiving HIV care.

Organizations indicated that housing services were scarce in Alameda
County, and there was an unmet need for more permanent housing options
in San Francisco. Overwhelmingly, across all organizations, housing emerged
as one of the biggest needs. As one interviewee noted:

> People are asking for . . . permanent housing that they can afford, permanent
> housing that is not . . . at some points where you'd not want to live in . . . More
> opportunities for shelter plus care. More opportunities for project indepen-
> dence, or . . . section 8 housing, but ways . . . for folks to access those types of
> housing. —Org. A

Many organizations also included drug use treatment, mental health treatment, and dental and vision services as additional health-related services that
clients frequently needed. Organizations that worked primarily with clients
in the city of San Francisco praised the availability of HIV medical and social
services, while those that worked in Alameda County (specifically, the city of
Oakland) noted a severe lack of services: "In Alameda County vs. SF County,
Alameda doesn't have the systems, the services, the system in terms of data
management, in terms of getting people into care, in terms of case management, centers of excellence, and all the things. So it really is a stark contrast"
(Org. B).

At the program level, organizations expressed several needs. Some relayed
the need for more education about HIV, including transmission prevention

for PLWH and community-level education to dispel misinformation and combat stigma. Organizations also reported the need for additional staff dedicated to linkage to care. As one respondent explained: "So . . . for us, we could easily have another [linkage coordinator's name] or two in addition to trying to have additional monies for our peers. So, there are, definitely, oodles of work to go around but not enough resources to cover the need" (Org. A).

In summary, across all organizations, housing emerged as a client need for which the availability of service did not meet the demand. Organizations working in San Francisco indicated that their clients had access to most of the HIV medical and social services they needed, while organizations working in Alameda County reported a severe lack of services. All organizations also indicated a need for additional staff to conduct linkage-to-care work. Respondents discussed this both in terms of the amount of time and effort needed to link highly marginalized clients to care and as a reflection of the number of PLWH who needed to be linked to care.

Overarching Conclusions

The BANPH project successfully linked an underserved population—individuals who faced many barriers—to ongoing medical care. Many factors contributed to this success, including addressing clients' most urgent needs (e.g., services for homelessness, mental health, and substance use). Providing these services also boosted client engagement. Small incentives for visits also helped. Relationships among BANPH partners helped with client referrals. Strong relationships between staff and clients were also seen as a key factor driving successful linkage to care.

According to the network analysis, organizations showed an increase in connectedness through PC, based on increased density score. Before PC, there were fewer connections, and the lead agency was responsible for most of these. However, interviews during the PC project suggested that although organizations were connected, it was not to the extent that they sought. Increasing MoUs and formal collaborations may alleviate these issues and allow easier sharing of client information.

BANPH faced some challenges to implementation of the program. Across the board, housing posed one of the toughest barriers to care, especially given the geographic context. Another difficulty was that individuals residing in Alameda County did not have access to nearly as many social services as

San Francisco residents. Organizations that worked with jails and prisons described challenges in navigating those systems. BANPH sought out the most underserved clients, which increased the challenges because of the burden of need faced by these clients, such as substance use, mental health issues, poverty, homelessness, and pervasive stigma.

Multiple Regions in the State of North Carolina

Background

In 2009, North Carolina had the eighth-highest rate of HIV diagnoses among the U.S. states at 23.8 per 100,000 and the eleventh-highest rate of AIDS diagnoses at 11.2 per 100,000 (Foust and Clymore 2011). In 2011, there were an estimated 25,607 adults and adolescents living with HIV in North Carolina. The total number of new HIV diagnoses in the state in 2010 was 1,487 (a rate of 15.9 per 100,000) (Centers for Disease Control and Prevention 2012a). Among these newly diagnosed cases of HIV, 26% of individuals were simultaneously diagnosed with AIDS or late presentation of HIV (Foust and Clymore 2011). From the beginning of the HIV epidemic to the end of 2010, North Carolina reported 38,397 HIV cases (Foust and Clymore 2011).

The distribution of HIV cases in North Carolina highlights the disproportionate effect on various segments of the population. For example, the highest rate of new HIV diagnoses was among adult/adolescent Black/African American males, with new diagnosis rates more than ten times those of their White counterparts. Black/African Americans (66% of all cases) and men (76% of all cases) are disproportionally affected by HIV. While 77 percent of new diagnoses in 2010 were in urban areas, some of the highest HIV disease rates were found in rural areas, especially among Black/African Americans and Hispanics (Foust and Clymore 2011).

A total of 246,458 persons were tested through state-sponsored HIV testing programs in 2010. Since 2004, the North Carolina Communicable Disease Branch (CDB) has administered a rapid testing program with funding from both federal and state sources. The nontraditional testing site program is also overseen by the CDB to serve underserved populations. Most HIV testing in North Carolina takes place in STI clinics, but other testing sites include emergency departments, community health centers, and corrections facilities (Foust and Clymore 2011).

In 2009, roughly 20 percent of the state's population aged 19 to 64 years was uninsured (Foust 2011 and Clymore). For people living with HIV (PLWH) in 2009, Medicaid was the most common type of insurance (39%), followed by Medicare (30%), and private insurance (30%); 19% of PLWH in North Carolina had no health insurance at some time during the previous 12-month period (Foust 2011 and Clymore).

North Carolina received $71,568,919 in federal HIV and AIDS funding in 2010. The federal total included $54,572,289 in Ryan White funding and $11,096,177 in Centers for Disease Control and Prevention HIV and AIDS funding. The remainder came from Housing Opportunities for Persons with AIDS (HOPWA), Substance Abuse and Mental Health Services Administration, and Office of Minority Health HIV/AIDS funding. Of the total HIV and AIDS funding in the state, $53,945,002 went to the AIDS Drugs Assistance Program (ADAP). In 2010, ADAP in North Carolina served 6,591 individuals with an estimated monthly cost of $832 per individual (Foust and Clymore 2011; NASTAD 2012). In 2013, the state provided $20 million through ADAP (NASTAD 2012).

Program Overview

Positive Charge (PC) in North Carolina was a collaboration of five organizations that sought to reach and serve PLWH across the state who were not engaged in medical care. The five organizations were spread across three geographic regions, and PC supported two or three access coordinators (ACs) in each region. The ACs worked directly with PLWH. Their role varied with the organization but could include conducting outreach, meeting with PLWH to encourage them to seek care, linking them to support services, and accompanying them to doctor's appointments. ACs are peers who often provide a healthy example of living with HIV.

Three geographic regions participated in the North Carolina PC program: rural northeastern, coastal southeastern, and Mecklenburg County. Each region had separate needs and strategies and hence largely worked independently. The Center for Health Policy and Inequalities Research at Duke University (CHPIR), the lead agency, worked collaboratively with its partners in these three regions.

Positive Charge Partner Organizations

The PC network in North Carolina comprised five organizations, as described below, collaborating to link PLWH to care in the three network regions: rural northeastern, suburban coastal, and urban Charlotte / Mecklenburg County area.

1. *The Center for Health Policy and Inequalities Research at Duke University (CHPIR)*: CHPIR was a key organizer of what began as a statewide collaboration of funders to support innovative HIV programs in North Carolina. The collaborators included the National AIDS Fund, Kate B. Reynolds Foundation, Duke Endowment, North Carolina Blue Cross Blue Shield Foundation, and Health and Wellness Trust Fund. This started in 2008 in recognition of a need for statewide approaches to HIV that would boost communities' capacity to improve the health of PLWH and individuals at risk for HIV. CHPIR continues to provide grants to a broadly defined group of grantees that provide prevention and care services. CHPIR also hosts National AIDS Fund AmeriCorps members who work with local organizations on HIV education, prevention, and care services.

As the lead organization in the PC initiative, CHPIR offered funding, resources, and leadership within the HIV prevention and care community. CHPIR coordinated communication between project partners and provided training and resources for the ACs.

2. *Hertford County Public Health Authority (HCPHA)*: HCPHA is the regional health authority responsible for a wide range of community health programs in eleven counties. HCPHA's community health priorities include preconception health, obesity, chronic disease, and AIDS. HCPHA is the lead agency in the local HIV network of care; it is the only agency providing HIV care in the region. As part of its work with the North Carolina PC network, HCPHA also used a mobile health unit, called "health in motion," to reach individuals living in rural surrounding areas. Activities conducted by the mobile unit included CD4 and viral load measurement and, two weeks later, medical advice to returning clients through a physician focusing on HIV. The health-in-motion units visited five sites. HCPHA also received referrals from the hospital emergency room and other organizations. It conducted outreach and provided services such as case management to out-of-care PLWH.

3. *Mecklenburg County Health Department (MCHD):* MCHD works to promote public health in Mecklenburg County through a variety of services for adults and children. It provides clinical and community services, including HIV counseling and testing, a sexually transmitted infection (STI) control clinic, Women, Infants and Children (WIC) services, pediatric dental services, HIV case management, communicable disease control, HIV/STI investigation, HIV community testing and outreach, and Ryan White services. As part of the North Carolina PC network, MCHD conducted testing within the community and found PC clients through referrals. MCHD's case managers worked to link out-of-care individuals to care and conducted laboratory testing (viral loads and CD4 counts).

4. *Regional AIDS Interfaith Network (RAIN, Inc.):* RAIN was founded in 1992 by Rev. Deborah Warren and a group of volunteers with the purpose of engaging the faith community in working with PLWH. RAIN offers holistic, direct services to members of all age groups living with HIV. Its range of services includes advocacy, pastoral counseling, education programs, and support groups. As part of the North Carolina PC, RAIN's access coordinators worked in the urban areas of Charlotte and greater Mecklenburg County to support clients before and after linkage to care and collaborated with local social services organizations to link clients with support services they needed.

5. *AIDS Care and Educational Services, Inc. (ACES):* ACES was founded in 1993 with the mission of administering Ryan White and HOPWA funds to benefit people living with HIV and AIDS in six North Carolina counties. In the PC project, ACES located out-of-care individuals and provided services to PLWH. For services not provided by ACES, such as dental care, ACES provided referrals. (ACES dissolved after data collection for this case study was completed.)

Tables 11 and 12 summarize the characteristics of the North Carolina PC network partners and the services they provided.

North Carolina Positive Charge Network
Network Graphic

Figure 10 represents the North Carolina PC network. Organizations are represented by boxes. The gray boxes across the top indicate the role each organization played in the linkage-to-care continuum: identification of PLWH who were out of care, linkage to care, provision of HIV primary care, and

Table 11 Positive Charge network partners, North Carolina

Organization	Legal fiscal designation	Type of health service agency	Annual HIV operation budget	Number of PLWH served, 2010	Number of paid employees, 2010	Number of volunteers, 2010
CHPIR	Private nonprofit	Not a health service agency	$600,000	n/a	1.5	0
HCPHA	Public	Local county/city/ state health department	$585,000	155	60–65	4–8
MCHD	Public	Local county/city/ state health department.	$45,441,760	n/a	~460	n/a
RAIN	Private nonprofit	AIDS service organization	$1,161,369	532	16	400
ACES	Public	AIDS service organization	$614,074	273	4	20

Note: All organization names are given in full in the text. n/a = not applicable.

Table 12 Services offered to PLWH by PC partner organizations

Organization	STI/HIV counseling and testing	HIV primary care	HIV case management	HIV outreach and linkage to care	HIV peer support	Other health services	Counseling services	HIV education and prevention services	Assistance with entitlement services	Support services*
HCPHA	×	×	×	×	×	×	×	×	×	H, T, N, S
MCHD	×		×	×	×			×		
RAIN				×	×			×		
ACES	×	×	×	×	×	×	×	×		

Note: CHPIR is not a direct service provider (it funds and coordinates work through other North Carolina AIDS service organizations) and therefore is not included in the table. All organization names are given in full in the text.

*H = housing; N = nutritional support or food; S = substance use treatment; T = transportation.

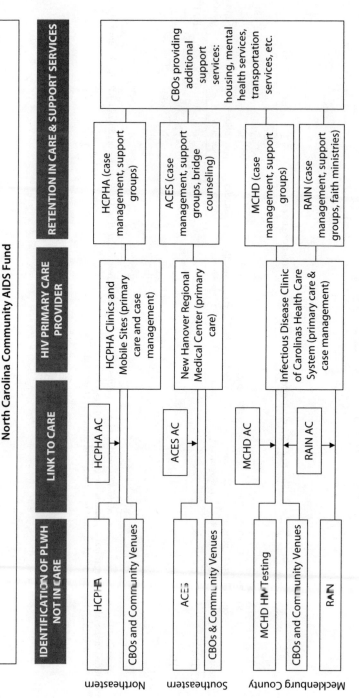

Figure 10. North Carolina Positive Charge network graphic

provision of support services. As represented by the long box at the top of the figure, CHPIR was the lead agency for PC in North Carolina and oversaw and coordinated the linkage-to-care activities.

Rural northeastern (eleven counties)

In the rural northeast, out-of-care PLWH were referred to HCPHA by health agencies such as the hospital emergency room. HCPHA also recruited program participants through outreach efforts at colleges, jails, and other locations. Some clients self-referred after hearing of HCPHA's services. After a client was located, usually through CAREWare (open-source Health Resources and Services Administration (HRSA)–sponsored software for managing HIV and AIDS care service data), a medical case manager at HCPHA worked to link the client to care and notified ACs if a client dropped out of care; the ACs located individuals who had dropped out of care. HCPHA provided care and support for some individuals, particularly those in rural areas, and used a mobile clinic unit. HCPHA's primary partners in its region included hospitals, doctors, and health departments.

Suburban coastal southeastern (six counties)

ACES initially located out-of-care PLWH through a CAREWare-generated list of names obtained from New Hanover Regional Medical Center. Many current ACES clients referred friends. Local community-based organizations (CBOs), several of which had Ryan White–funded case managers, also referred clients to ACES. Once a client was referred, another ACES staff member referred the client for case management and medical care. ACs worked to find out-of-care individuals and link them to care and support services. ACES also provided a variety of support services, and clients were referred for other services such as eye care and dental services.

Urban Charlotte / Mecklenburg County

In Mecklenburg County, where the urban center of Charlotte is located, MCHD and RAIN worked together to link, retain, and support individuals living with HIV. RAIN engaged individuals primarily through community outreach by ACs. Local shelters and home care agencies also referred individuals. RAIN ACs were often peers and performed a wide variety of functions to support clients before and after linkage to care. While they could not provide case management, ACs could accompany clients to doctor's visits and conduct support groups. RAIN also worked with several local CBOs, pharmacies, and churches to link clients to support services.

MCHD enrolled new clients who were identified through testing in the community or referred by county disease intervention services, as well as individuals soon to be released from jail. Primary care providers also referred individuals to MCHD. MCHD-based case managers worked with the newly enrolled clients and involved ACs to follow up with them. ACs linked clients to support services, including peer support groups and drug assistance programs. MCHD also had an in-house nurse practitioner who conducted CD4 and viral load tests but could not prescribe medication. MCHD ACs and case managers worked closely together throughout the process.

Network Sociogram

We used UCINET (Borgatti et al. 2002) to assess the ties between organizations and the change in ties following implementation of PC. Sites were asked which PC partners they currently worked with and whether they had worked with PC partners to link PLWH to care in the six months before the start of the project. These two questions allowed a comparison between the linkage-to-care networks before and after the start of the PC.

Figure 11 is a sociogram of the linkage-to-care network in North Carolina during the PC project. The density of the PC network was 0.80, meaning 16 ties out of a possible 20. The average degree, or number of connections per organization, was 3.2. The network centralization was 17%, representing the extent to which one organization accounted for all of the network connections.

Figure 12 shows the sociogram six months before PC was implemented. The network had a density of only 0.40, an average degree of 1.4, and a network centralization score of 17%. Thus, following implementation of the PC project, network centralization stayed the same, but the density doubled from 0.40 to 0.80. Coupled with the unchanged network centralization score, the increase in density score suggests an overall increase in collaboration among organizations. Visual examination of the two sociograms supports these observations. Before PC, there were two distinct groups of organizations. Through the course of PC, these disparate organizations gained connections.

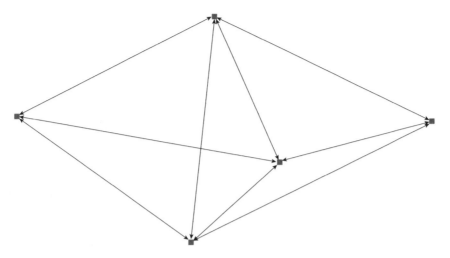

Figure 11. North Carolina Positive Charge network sociogram

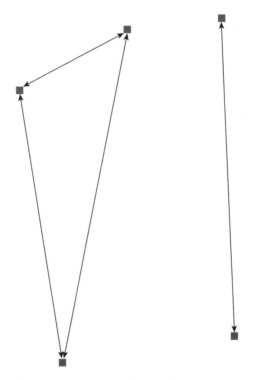

Figure 12. North Carolina organizational network sociogram six months before
Positive Charge

Internal Structural Changes

All partner organizations reported beneficial changes resulting from PC. Of particular note were the addition of new positions—the ACs—within the organizations and the expansion of services.

ACs were able to fit easily into existing systems. A respondent explained: "They've [ACs] kind of fit into the existing system except for the fact that when a referral is made now, they're an additional person that's being told about the particular client coming into care" (Org. C). In a few instances, there was a period of adjustment when the role of the ACs within the organization was not clear. One AC recounted: "We also had to let them [the organization] know what our roles were because they thought they were going to dump off a whole lot more on us" (Org. D). The AC explained that this relationship was quickly ironed out, and the case managers now appreciated having the ACs to call on to support their clients. Case managers noted that ACs—who shared experiences with clients—were better able to relate to and engage clients.

Several organizations offered support groups and community education after PC began. An administrator explained that "[ACs are] going out and being part of the support groups; going out to the community; being able to talk to people one on one; not having to adhere to the state guidelines . . . just having a little bit more freedom in what you're doing" (Org. A).

The ACs were also able to fill gaps in the organizations, helping to complete tasks that were previously left uncompleted. For example, an individual reported: "The AC could make those appointments for the early intervention clinic directly and then could meet those individuals, could even transport them to a clinic appointment or meet them here, and I know that's helped with some of the no-show rate" (Org. D).

One organization (Org. B) was undergoing structural changes related to changes in leadership and loss of government funding streams (Ryan White and Medicaid). In the past it had offered case management services, but changes to North Carolina's endorsement system for case managers caused the organization to drop case management because, under the new guidelines, it would no longer be financially feasible. According to one AC:

> [The organization] is reconstructing itself. Changing the mission; we're pretty much becoming a direct service type of organization for individuals living with HIV and AIDS, so PC right now is fitting perfectly because we're outreach-

ing to the individuals who know their status who are not in care and getting them into care. —Org. B

In this way, becoming part of the PC project helped guide the focus of the organization's restructuring.

Identification of Clients

For a few partner organizations, identification of out-of-care PLWH, at least initially, was the most challenging aspect of linkage to care. The biggest difficulty was lack of access to the names of people who were out of care. The health department's disease intervention specialists (DIS) generate a list of PLWH who are out of care through CAREWare. The ACs at one organization worked for almost a year to gain access to the list generated through CARE-Ware at the large nearby hospital. Once they had access to CAREWare, the job of identification became much easier: "I get into CAREWare now and pull up a list of new names every two weeks and we go over the list . . . and go from there" (Org. B). One respondent thought initially that the organization would be getting more information from DIS, but found that "the cooperation on that level has not been there" (Org. B).

Agencies in other locations found that the cooperation of DIS was crucial in their ability to identify people who needed linkage to care. One respondent reported that "we work with the DIS . . . [DIS] will call us and actually let us talk to the client and set their first appointment" (Org. C). Another respondent also described getting referrals from DIS: "DIS is a source. They allow us to know who's tested positive in the community" (Org. D).

For all partner organizations in North Carolina, referrals were an important method of locating people who needed linkage to care. Many organizations received informal referrals from other organizations working in the area. For example, one agency (Org. B) received referrals from a local men's shelter and a home care agency. It seems that these exchanges of client information took place either within one system (e.g., the department of public health) or within the confines of a memorandum of exchange (MoU). The need to exchange client information in locating underserved individuals underscores the importance of MoUs that allow this type of information sharing and of clear guidelines within organizations about what client information can and cannot be shared. One AC described the challenges of working without easy access to client information:

Someone tests positive and then they [providers] can't tell you the person's positive so you can help them. It's not like we want to hurt them. We want to let them know about our services. Sometimes it seems like . . . they're hurting the clients more than helping them because it ends up sometimes becoming an issue because you can't find out what you need to know to help the client. —Org. C

In addition to formal and informal referrals from partnering organizations, referrals came from a variety of sources. Current and former clients often referred people they knew who could benefit from the services offered by PC. Friends and family members sometimes referred people because they had heard about the program through word of mouth.

Outreach and support groups were other methods used to recruit into the PC program. The ACs at one organization (Org. B) in particular had a lot of previous experience with outreach and advocacy. When their collaboration with the health department did not go as expected, they shifted their focus to outreach and education activities. According to one AC, they went to "churches, barbershops, beauty salons, parks, whatever. It doesn't matter" (Org. B). When another organization (Org. A) initially had trouble accessing the list of people who had dropped out of care, it began to offer support groups. Through these groups, Org. A staff were able to engage program participants.

Finally, testing and contacting people newly diagnosed with HIV was a successful strategy for identification. One organization reported that it frequently took its mobile unit out for education or testing events. Food and music were often included as a draw. "This week alone we did the . . . community college and we had 30 people come out and get tested" (Org. C).

Outreach and Linkage to Care

To understand the linkage-to-care landscape before the PC project, we asked each organization to describe how linkage to care was conducted prior to PC. None of the organizations reported doing more than minimal linkage to care. Even these minimal efforts were hampered by lack of staffing and structure. One site described its previous approach as "passive", it would make referrals if asked. Another site reported that it made an effort to provide linkage to care but that it was "hectic" and done only on an ad hoc basis by volunteers. One respondent described how the approach to linkage to care had changed now that the organization was part of PC: "It used to be one guy doing it 25%, and now we've got three guys who do it more full time and maybe are also using other techniques because they have the time to be able to do that" (Org. C).

PC linkage-to-care specialists used a variety of strategies to contact PC clients, including phone calls, home visits, and personal contact at testing events or support groups. Sites reiterated that taking the time to fully understand clients' needs and concerns was critical for building rapport and establishing trust. For peers, sharing their own story and listening to the stories of their clients was another important step in building a relationship and establishing credibility. Across all sites, it was understood that while getting clients into care was the ultimate goal, clients' basic life needs had to be addressed first. Therefore, relationship building and addressing barriers to care were key components of linkage to care:

> It's important to identify what's bothering people because . . . that can lead to forgetting to take the medications. —Org. C

> I ask them on the intake form, "What are the things that you have need of?" or "What's the most important service?" so right then I can make a referral for them to get food, and sometimes when they leave they can go to that location and pick up food. That helps to get everything that they need right then. And then we go forward. —Org. B

In North Carolina, providers reported that housing, substance use, and unemployment were the most pressing concerns for PC clients. In addition, many clients needed general support and motivation in areas of life not addressed by case managers, who focused solely on medical issues.

Once a client was ready to be linked to care, PC linkage-to-care workers facilitated the linkage through a variety of strategies, such as making appointments, arranging or providing transportation, giving appointment reminders, and attending lab and clinic appointments with clients. Some sites worked closely with case managers and bridge counselors. At one site, identification, linkage, HIV care, and follow-up were all done through a mobile health unit. ACs often continued to work with their clients through phone calls, home visits, and transportation arrangements and by accompanying them to appointments until barriers to care had been addressed and clients were established in a regular system of care. As one AC put it: "My goal for them is to be self-sufficient and not depend so much on you" (Org. D). However, sites appreciated the freedom to continue working with clients as long as they needed support.

Facilitators of PC Implementation

Peer-to-peer support was by far the most frequently mentioned facilitating factor. Both administrators and ACs felt that the shared experiences of the coordinators enabled them to relate to clients in a way that other service providers could not. As one AC put it: "It's the peer aspect, the fact that you're a peer and that you can be a mentor because you've gone through it . . . I've been [living with HIV] 18 years; I'm still here and you can't even tell" (Org. C). The fact that ACs were often individuals living with HIV was inspiring to clients who feared the long-term health consequences from their illness.

The peers could also provide information about firsthand experiences with treatment, medication, and medical providers that case managers and other service providers could not. This peer aspect was seen, across the board, as the most valuable aspect of the PC program:

> It definitely has impacted the other services. Like, we try to do an assessment of clients when they first come in to care with us, but sometimes clients won't tell us everything up front because they don't fully trust you, but the ACs, when they talk with them, a lot of times they're more open with them, so they [clients] may end up in some cases telling them things they may not have told us about, so they [ACs] can kind of help persuade them. —Org. C

Another facilitating factor was the partnerships that some organizations had already established before PC. An administrator noted:

> For a health department it's going to be most important to work out those partnerships with the local DIS and make sure that you got clear communication with the testing program at the clinic or an outreach for testing program . . . Already having an established partnership with an infectious disease clinic makes it much easier being a part of the hospital system. I don't think [any other North Carolina PC site] has that kind of situation in trying to go ahead and set up that partnership. —Org. D

Finally, having personal passion for the job and working for an organization with an established reputation in the community were mentioned as factors that contributed to the success of PC.

Organizations reported that PC had enabled most partner organizations to expand services and serve more PLWH. All the organizations mentioned that PC's flexibility, compared with other funders, enabled a more creative approach. PC's commitment to "learning" was also noted; an administrator appreciated that participation in the project had been a comfortable and collaborative process.

Unmet Client Needs and Barriers to PC Implementation

Respondents reported a number of factors that presented barriers to implementation of the PC program and to clients' participation.

Transportation

The barrier mentioned most frequently was transportation for both clients and access coordinators. ACs had to travel to locate clients and sometimes provided transportation to appointments. Two sites (Org. A and Org. C) were located in areas where the population of PLWH and the sites that provided services to them were very spread out. Reaching clients and getting them to their medical appointments could be difficult and time consuming. A respondent (Org. A) spoke of clients in one county who had to travel to another county for services, a round trip of 160 miles. One AC described the transportation problem as follows:

> You're looking at very rural counties and we have to cover all that area, and one of our sites, from here it takes us 2 hours to get there and some places maybe longer. It's definitely the travel and the cost of transportation to go see clients, so to follow up with people if you're trying to find somebody, to get to their house. —Org. C

Several respondents mentioned that ACs used their own vehicles, putting significant mileage on their cars often without reimbursement for wear and tear or even full coverage for fuel costs. While most sites allowed their ACs to transport clients, one did not (Org. C). The AC felt that this added to clients' burden.

Shortage of support services

Organizations indicated shortages in a variety of support services for PLWH, including mental health and substance use treatment and job placement, food, heating fuel, and housing assistance. For example, one site (Org. C) estimated that around 90% of its clients were unemployed and needed job training. On addressing basic needs, one respondent explained: "One of our biggest issues right now in the substance abuse area is the fact that people go into treatment and they have nowhere to go . . . You have to get your basic needs met first. That's true across the board" (Org. B).

Medical providers

More medical providers, including primary care providers, infectious disease specialists, and dentists, were needed for PLWH. In Mecklenburg County, agencies (Org. B and Org. D) faced a lack of providers, particularly for uninsured patients. Two respondents commented on the general provider problem:

> It could be six weeks before we can even get them in to see a case manager. There were no Ryan White providers that were taking any new patients, and that periodically happens. We're scrambling to find somebody who can take someone in. —Administrator, Org. D

> Right now we're having to commute to Concord to get somebody into care. In some instances, we have [a nurse practitioner] at the Health department who will write a prescription initially, but we have to find doctors. —AC, Org. B

Staffing needs

Additional case managers in rural areas would provide better services to clients and potentially alleviate some of the transportation burden on clients and ACs.

Training

An administrator noted the need to create a more comprehensive training program to train ACs not only for PC sites but for other organizations and agencies that were looking to hire peers. Adequate, ongoing training was needed, particularly for ACs who joined after the start of the project.

Centralized services

Sites reported the need for more centralized services for PLWH. An administrator explained: "Mental health is separate from substance abuse which is separate . . . there's not that much social support, and most of those have been taken on by individual consumers, so there's not a lot of agencies that are doing multiple services" (Org. D).

Support groups

Several organizations noted a need for additional facilitated support groups that met regularly because, for PLWH, "if you have no one else to talk to, you need that reinforcement" (Org. C). Service providers saw support groups as important elements for retention and cited the need for support groups that could meet at times convenient to clients or that would serve particular populations.

Unsuccessful collaboration

Problematic relationships with other organizations and within partner organizations were also seen as a significant barrier. Several partner organizations reported that they wished the relationships between PC and DIS and care providers had been established before the project began. Several PC partners expended significant energy trying to partner with DIS or providers. In one case (Org. A), efforts to work with a local medical center and gain access to CAREWare eventually paid off. In another case (Org. B), attempts to work with a group of providers had not yet succeeded, despite initial provider enthusiasm at a providers' meeting (organized by Org. B).

Bureaucracy was seen as a culprit in preventing organizations from working together and in keeping information from PC partners. This was also seen within organizations when ACs found it difficult to get permission from their supervisors or those "higher up" to do things they thought would benefit their clients. One example was the frustration expressed by ACs who wanted to increase their visibility in the community:

> We created a website; we wanted to do a Facebook page. We also wanted to do Twitter; I did compile all this information; also created a brochure, but we still have not gotten approval yet. I know it takes time . . . but it has to go to so many different chains . . . they never allow us to get more visibility in the community so people know we exist. —Org. D

An administrator described initial push-back from established AIDS service organizations that feared the PC-funded organizations/agencies would take their clients. Efforts were made to inform these organizations that the intent of PC was to fill gaps and complement existing programs. While these efforts somewhat alleviated the resistance and mistrust, they were not completely ameliorated.

Policy

When asked about policy, respondents considered how their organizations were affected by both national policies and internal, organizational policies. Several sites reported frustration with how HIPAA (Health Insurance Portability and Accountability Act) privacy and confidentiality policies made it more difficult to identify and assist some clients. However, even those who expressed this frustration were quick to add that they supported the policy and knew that it couldn't be changed: "Unfortunately the biggest policy hurdle we have is a necessary one and that's protecting the patient's privacy and confidentiality. I wouldn't change it" (Org. D). This respondent's site went on to suggest that one way to overcome some of the limitations of HIPAA would be to involve providers in getting their patients to supply release-of-information documentation.

Another common source of frustration was national funding policies. One theme that emerged was how HRSA funds are distributed based on historical rates of HIV and AIDS, which allocates more funding to New York and California:

> We see growing rates [of HIV and AIDS] in the southeast; we don't see as much funding as we'd like to see. I know that some federal agencies have been readjusting that formula and looking at current incidence rates, and it would be great if HRSA did that. —Org. D

> I think there's a real disparity in the amount of funding some areas get versus what we get in the South. Right here in our county there's absolutely very minimal dental care, but if you're positive and you live in another community, NY, CA, or wherever, you have access to so many more services because of the way formularies are set up. —Org. B

Ryan White funding restrictions were also mentioned by several sites. Once a budget is set, it is difficult to change, even if client needs differ from what was anticipated:

> If we see that clients need more substance abuse counseling, sometimes you can't foresee that kind of stuff up front, and if you've got x amount of dollars in that line [item] to spend but you're already at it [that limit], and you've got five people that need to be seen and you know that will push you over, but they don't want you to spend what you have in that line, so then you have to hold off or overspend and deal with it later, which sometimes happens. —Org. C

Limitations on the number of times a client could be seen were also criticized: "Everybody's going to be different" (Org. B). Recent changes in how North Carolina certifies case management agencies were mentioned by more than one site but had a big impact on one site (Org. B) in particular: "The requirement for having agencies that provide case management services be authorized to take Medicaid, which means they're going to have to get through certification. That's impossible for a small service organization. They're not going to be able to do that" (Org B). As a result, this PC site stopped providing case management services: "We decided that we couldn't afford to go through the process."

Internal organizational polices were also mentioned. One site did not allow ACs to transport clients. This caused a lot of frustration for ACs, who felt they could be more effective at getting people into care if they were able to transport them to their appointments. One AC noted: "When I was able to transport, that's when I was really successful. I get my hands on [a client], I'm not letting [the client] go until I get [him/her] here. But [my supervisor] said I can't do that" (Org. C). One site reported feeling restricted by internal policies on marketing. A proposal to increase marketing had been submitted months ago but was slow to move through the internal bureaucracy.

Finally, policy was also mentioned in a positive way. One site noted that clear policies helped people understand their roles and limitations. An AC from another site, referring to the perceived lack of bureaucracy in her agency, said: "I love our policy because we go to the CEO and she says, 'Yes'" (Org. B).

Overarching Conclusions

Participation in the PC project in North Carolina was associated with increased organizational capacity and reach. Access coordinators were credited with much of the project's success because they were able to engage with clients in a way that case managers previously could not. Despite initial challenges in integrating ACs into project activities, the additional bandwidth offered by these new staff members allowed organizations to provide more services to more clients.

Individual organizations were more connected to one another after implementation of PC, as evidenced by the increased network density. Qualitative interviews suggested that this may have been due in part to informal connections among individuals at implementing agencies. This idea is further supported by the network analysis, which found no increase in network centralization during PC, meaning that all actors were equally connected to others; no single coordinating body emerged. The organizations most successful in linkage to HIV care were those that formed successful partnerships.

Several environmental factors remained challenges for successful linkage and retention in care that must be addressed by state and national policy. These challenges included a lack of available providers, even in urban areas, and restrictions on the use of Ryan White funds. Another factor cited as key for success was referrals between organizations to identify out-of-care PLWH. Future programs should continue to proactively establish MoUs to allow referral of clients or use client release forms to appropriately share client information.

Linkage-to-care programs should be designed to address barriers to care such as transportation and other unmet client needs. Programs should include a significant, integrated support service component, including basic client needs such as transportation to appointments, mental health care, housing and job placement services, and substance use treatment.

Overall, PC program staff were enthusiastic about the success of the program, particularly peers, who wished they had had peer support, in addition to case management, when they were first diagnosed with HIV:

> I think it's an awesome program. When I was diagnosed . . . I wish it was around for me. [There] was a lot more money around then so I was able to get the case management services. But when the case load started to fill up, you were pushed to the side because it was a lot on the case managers. So just having peer support to assist with individual[s] that are diagnosed with HIV and AIDS, it's a plus, and they [peers] help them [clients] to move towards living more and how to navigate the system . . . to take care of themselves. —Org. D

Conclusions

Summary of Findings

This volume describes an embedded multiple-case study of five individual Positive Charge (PC) programs. Across all sites, many PC implementation experiences were shared. Almost all sites hired additional staff to conduct linkage-to-care activities and increased their organizations' focus on linkage to care. Sites also reported increased collaboration across partner agencies, which proved to be both beneficial and challenging. For some sites, working with clinical partners was particularly difficult. All sites reported that unmet client needs had to be addressed before linkage-to-care work could proceed. Housing, in particular, emerged as a dire need. Clients also faced significant psychosocial barriers to care, such as distrust of the medical system. And finally, programs had difficulty locating clients because their contact information changed often.

Several implementation experiences were significant but not shared across all sites. At the system level, these experiences included challenges in navigating systems such as jails and prisons, lack of transportation, and lack of adequate social support services. Growing partnerships and working with local partner organizations also unfolded differently for each site. Within the PC network, one site desired deeper collaboration with its partners, and another found that formalized learning sessions helped its project. Organizationally, some sites had to develop new techniques for identification and linkage, while other sites had more experience in this area. Similarly, some sites struggled with data management, reporting, and staff turnover, while others did not report these challenges.

Factors aiding linkage included emphasizing the relationship between clients and linkage workers and using client incentives. Sites working with peers credited them with the program's success and lauded their passion and dedication.

However, these sites had to mitigate tension caused by role confusion between the duties of peers and those of case managers. Other challenges included learning and maintaining appropriate professional boundaries and investing in initial training. Nonetheless, the PC sites unequivocally praised peers' work with clients.

Experiences with Linkage to Care

The five PC programs had very different experiences with initial recruitment. Across all sites, successful strategies included having HIV testing services available in-house and linking newly diagnosed individuals to care; obtaining referrals from a variety of organizations that worked with newly diagnosed individuals, including providers; scanning lists of partner organizations' clients and contacting those who were lost to care; reaching out-of-care individuals upon their admission to a hospital; conducting outreach on the street and in the community; and peers seeking new clients through their networks. For incarcerated populations, meeting potential clients before or immediately after release was very important for retention in the program. Sites that did not have lists of out-of-care people living with HIV (PLWH) found it challenging to recruit eligible participants. Although the lists eased finding out-of-care individuals, making contact with individuals on the list still proved challenging for all organizations. One linkage-to-care worker explained that, on a list, "I have seen a total of 46 to start with . . . I weed it down . . . to 25 and from those 25 I found . . . about 9." Contact information, such as cellphone numbers and emergency contacts, are frequently out of date.

Two sites had unique advantages in locating and recruiting individuals. In the PC network in Louisiana (PC Louisiana), the statewide Louisiana Public Health Information Exchange list was available to the local PC program through close collaboration with the disease intervention services. It proved to be vital in identifying out-of-care PLWH. Similarly, in New York City's network (PC New York), Amida Care was a managed care organization that simply analyzed medical claims data to identify out-of-care individuals.

Across all sites, strategies for establishing an initial linkage between client and clinic were very similar. All sites started by building rapport, addressing clients' individual needs, making a physician's appointment, and reminding clients about their appointments. Depending on the client's level of need, linkage workers might accompany the client to the first medical appointment. Several sites also provided transportation. Health navigators described how some clients preferred to meet outside their offices in more neutral locations (e.g., a local fast-food restaurant). Most sites also mentioned that this process was time consuming and varied greatly by client.

Collaboration across PC Networks

Evidence suggests that participation in PC boosted network connectedness. Across the four sites with data available, connectedness among network partners increased as measured by density, node degree, and network centralization scores (no network analysis was conducted for PC New York due to insufficient data). Density is the number of connections between organizations as a fraction of the total possible number of connections. Comparing density six months before PC and during PC, we found that this measurement increased at three of the four sites; the site that did not see an increase, the Chicago network (PC Chicago), already had the maximum possible density prior to PC. Node degree is simply the average number of connections per organization, and, across all sites, it was higher during than prior to PC. Network centralization scores characterize the extent to which a single organization is responsible for connections within a network. A lower network centralization score means that more organizations are directly connected to one another rather than through a single organization. In North Carolina's network (PC North Carolina) and PC Chicago, network centralization was the same before and during PC, while centralization decreased in the PC programs in the San Francisco / Bay Area (BANPH) and Louisiana.

Collaboration in PC networks was a challenging task for reasons specific to each site. In PC New York, network partners had high turnover, and some did not fully understand the roles of the community health outreach workers (CHOWs) and health navigators. This made it difficult for CHOWs and navigators to gain crucial client information from these network partners. PC Chicago's challenge was that partners thought members of the network often operated in silos. PC Louisiana and PC North Carolina both reported that collaborative working relationships formed slowly despite significant initial investment. BANPH and PC North Carolina both faced the difficulty of being unable to refer or share client information to the extent needed. Memoranda of understanding (MoUs) were not in place, or staff did not completely understand what was contained in the MoUs. Instead, sites that were not part of the same larger organization, such as county government, relied on information releases for individual clients. At BANPH and PC North Carolina, sharing information about who was eligible for Positive Charge was seen as extremely important to the program's success. Contacting eligible individuals whose names were on a clinic or local government list (in-reach) was very important for finding out-of-care PLWH.

Collaboration with clinical partners proved a unique challenge. For PC sites that did not have longstanding relationships with clinical partners, this collaboration was hard to establish. At smaller community-based organizations, health navigators collaborated with clinics but reported that some clinic staff were reluctant to proactively incorporate health navigation into their systems of service delivery. PC Chicago's respondents recommended securing MoUs proactively, and PC Louisiana's health navigators initiated conversations with providers to advocate for their work, a process that overcame initial resistance; some providers even referred their family members to PC.

On the whole, respondents were very enthusiastic about collaborating with their networks. In fact, the organizations most successful in locating and linking out-of-care individuals to HIV care were those that formed successful partnerships, often based on informal connections among individuals. All sites mentioned that PC had resulted in greater collaboration across network agencies and that this led to a wide variety of benefits for their PC programs. PC New York was the only site to participate in a formal, cross-organizational learning group, and several respondents mentioned that it was helpful. Other sites had informal cross-organizational sharing, and PC Louisiana's collaborations were so strong that partners stationed staff at each other's agencies. Louisiana's close collaborations benefited clients because a referral could be made to a specific individual, and services could be tailored to clients' needs (e.g., finding the clinic closest to the client). In PC North Carolina, network partnerships allowed multiple organizations to leverage the key, informal relationships across individuals who knew PLWH in their local communities.

Parallels across Sites' Implementation Experiences

At all five sites, access to "clean, decent, affordable housing" was repeatedly mentioned as a primary concern for clients and as a need that, when met, contributed greatly to successful engagement. Staff from all seven organizations interviewed as part of BANPH mentioned housing, and in PC New York, one participant estimated that more than 60% of clients needed housing assistance. In New York City and Louisiana, respondents described how challenging it was to navigate housing assistance programs. The PC Louisiana project emphasized that for incarcerated clients recently released, housing was often their primary concern.

All five sites also found there was a constellation of client needs that took precedence over HIV care. As one respondent at PC New York put it: "There are patients who are dealing with many other things, like not having a place to live, not having food, not having a job, and that interferes with their ability to make their health care a priority." The needs most often mentioned included substance use and mental health treatment and job placement services. Most sites also described overburdened social service systems that were not able to address all of these needs for clients in a way that was appropriate for them. BANPH saw addressing client needs as a way to nurture relationships with clients, and respondents at PC North Carolina suggested that collocated services would be the best way to address these client needs. In addition to basic needs, three sites described another set of difficult barriers: a variety of psychosocial barriers driven by stigma. A PC New York respondent described clients who initially did not see investing in their own health as worthwhile: "I don't want to go to the doctor" and "Who cares about me?" BANPH and PC Louisiana respondents also mentioned that there was a strong HIV-related stigma and clients often distrusted the medical system. In Louisiana, respondents mentioned that a strategy for mitigating these barriers was open communication with peers or health navigators, who shared their personal narrative of living with HIV.

Each site described significant changes in its organization during the PC program. The New York City, Chicago, North Carolina, and BANPH projects all described hiring additional staff. In fact, one PC New York agency combined other grant funding with PC funding to invest heavily in its linkage to care and retention in care. This organization increased the number of individuals in its Retention in Care department from one to twenty. BANPH was the only project with significant linkage-to-care experience prior to PC. Before PC, the majority of sites conducted linkage-to-care work on an ad hoc basis. As a PC Chicago respondent described, PC was the "first concerted effort to really identify and link newly diagnosed" individuals and "to identify folks who may have dropped out of care."

Several sites mentioned that a strong relationship between clients and linkage workers was critical to success. Incidentally, these were the same sites that used peer navigation as a strategy. For these sites, peers were largely credited for the success of the program. Peer roles did not come without challenges, however. Sites reported frustration resulting from confusion about the role of peers versus case managers, and peers did not always feel adequately supported in doing their jobs. Finally, each site attributed its success, in part, to tenacious, passionate, and dedicated linkage-to-care staff—particularly peers who could serve as examples and guides for their clients' journey from linkage to retention in care. A PC Louisiana respondent noted that "many clients have expressed that if it were not for him [the linkage worker] they would not be in care."

Differences across Sites

Each site mentioned the need for greater social support services for their clients. Transportation emerged as a dire need in PC Louisiana and PC North Carolina; this was strongly emphasized by linkage workers in these areas. PC Louisiana lacked reliable public transportation, while in the North Carolina program, there were often long driving times between clinics and clients' homes in rural areas. The sites located in major metropolitan areas did not struggle with the transportation issue to the same extent. PC New York was able to address this issue by providing public transportation passes, and BANPH used passes as client incentives. While PC Chicago mentioned challenges with transportation, it did not emerge as a major barrier to care.

All sites mentioned that clients' needs had to be addressed before linkage could occur and that meeting these various needs was challenging. More than the others, PC Louisiana and PC North Carolina emphasized repeatedly that social support services were lacking in their areas. Louisiana and North Carolina described a dire need for social support services for PLWH who were struggling with mental health issues, substance use, and job placement in addition to their other needs. BANPH had a hybrid situation in which social support services differed vastly depending on county of residence.

PC New York and PC Chicago both mentioned struggling with data management and timely reporting, but Chicago interviewees were grateful because, for the first time, the site was able to use data to prevent duplication of efforts and to influence their programmatic next steps.

Limitations of the Study

Several limitations are worthy of mention. The case studies used a descriptive methodology; hence, cause-and-effect relationships cannot be explored. Each case study is a snapshot of the PC grantee and its network at one point in time; it is not representative of the project as a whole or of the project at its completion. Organizations that were previously part of this grant could not be interviewed; only staff from partner organizations during the time of data collection could be interviewed. Due to time and funding limitations, we selected two individuals per organization for interview. A richer understanding may have resulted if we had gathered data from a broader swath of staff from each organization. Other individuals involved in the program may have held different perspectives that would have further enriched each case study. As a result, some information, details, and perspectives have most likely been omitted. While we tried to interview and survey at least two individuals from each organization in each site's network, we were not always able to do so, often due to scheduling constraints.

At each site, there were some organizations from which we were unable to interview a single individual. Also, many sites lacked survey data from several organizations. For sites with fewer surveys completed, we could not assess, in a network analysis, whether both organizations reported collaboration with each other. We could address only whether one organization reported collaboration with the other. For PC New York, so few organizations were surveyed that no network analysis was possible.

There are limitations when using online surveys. Previous research suggests that online surveys (when compared with more classical methods of data collection) may face issues such as missing data, unacceptable responses, and duplicate submissions (Schmidt 1997). However, we took steps in the survey design to mitigate these potential limitations. These steps included using short surveys with clear, concise language; using categorical or value-limited survey questions; and requiring completion of all questions. In the case of duplicate submissions, we used the most recent, and we did not use any unfinished survey responses. Several research studies suggest that data gathered through online surveys, when compared with classic modes of data collection, are equally valid and reliable (Deutskens et al. 2006; Krantz et al. 1997; Nathanson and Reinert 1999; Eysenbach and Wyatt 2002).

Because Positive Charge was devised and executed as a grant program with an evaluation component, the five sites were chosen based on a competitive proposal process. This process considered the local HIV epidemic but also the sites' ability to carry out linkage to care and retention in care successfully. As a result, some severely affected major metropolitan areas (e.g., Atlanta) were not part of PC. Furthermore, the HIV epidemic at each of the five PC locations has unique characteristics.

While these are indeed limitations of the study, the insights gained from the case studies, particularly the New Orleans (part of the Louisiana case study) and New York City programs, may be of use to other areas looking to do similar work in an urban context. We urge caution, however, about generalizing these findings to other geographies and organizations. The programs differ significantly and are affected by the needs and resources within their geographic locations. Other differences among sites may have affected the findings, such as the operations of the local and state health departments, available social services in each area, and other geography-specific characteristics such as housing markets and transportation options.

Recommendations

The five programs described in this book began at a time when there were few programs addressing the needs of PLWH who had never engaged in care or had dropped out of care. These five programs attempted this work when relatively few precedents existed; hence, their trailblazing experiences are valuable for future groups conducting similar work. By analyzing the experiences gained in these case studies, we compiled the following recommendations:

1. *Recognize and plan for a complex constellation of client needs:* As many site interviewees commented on the unexpected intensity of client needs and felt somewhat unprepared to address them, future programs could consider building adequate time and resources into their budgets and plans before the start of the program. Estimates of how long it will take to link a particular client into HIV care should reflect the time required for the client's outstanding needs to be met before linkage can occur.

2. *Nurture and cultivate interorganizational networks despite inevitable challenges:* While establishing a network of organizations proved challenging for each site, all reported strong, concrete benefits, including referrals or provision of social services needed by clients. Organizations found that their networks were strengthened by engaging partners as early in the program as possible and by seeking buy-in from senior management. Previous studies have found that collaboration begins through information sharing, followed by referrals, and finally, sharing of resources (Provan et al. 2003). Based on the experience of PC New York, it seems that formal learning communities or meetings may also aid in this process.

3. *Proactively establish procedures to share information about clients or potential clients:* Establishing relationships with organizations that had access to lists of out-of-care clients (e.g., local health departments) before beginning the PC project was found to benefit programs in starting the linkage process. Sites could also consider establishing MoUs early on, which could enable partners to share information about individuals that may be eligible for retention-in-care programs across partner organizations (e.g., between an AIDS service organization that does case management and clinical partners). MoUs have a distinct advantage in that they allow organizations to gain information on an individual before that individual is contacted. Client release forms also allow the sharing of client information between organizations while respecting confidentiality. This method does not aid initial client recruitment, however, because it requires contact with clients who may be challenging to locate initially.

4. *Create strong relationships with medical providers:* Sites lacking pre-existing relationships with medical providers should cultivate such relationships early in the program, using a variety of ways to connect with this vital group that often proves challenging to engage. Partnerships should be established as early as possible. Collocating case managers and linkage-to-care workers in clinical settings may provide an opportunity to accomplish this.

5. *Involve peers or other health navigators to support clients in linking to care:* All of the programs employing peers as linkage-to-care workers found the role of these workers to be vital to the success of the project. Previous studies reported similar findings; a variety of linkage workers can be successful (Bradford 2007; Thompson et al. 2012). Our findings suggest that creating a supportive, enabling work environment for peers could proactively address some common initial misunderstandings. Concrete steps could include providing peers with resources (e.g., office space) and clarifying peer roles versus case manager roles at the outset.

6. *Ongoing organizational management:* The experiences of the PC sites in our case studies suggest that ongoing organizational management issues such as staff and partner organization turnover pose a challenge to linkage-to-care programs. Suggestions could include addressing staff turnover, establishing back-up plans in case of absences or unanticipated staff changes, and offering training or mentorship for work in new areas (for staff new to computer use in a professional setting, staff new to prison systems, etc.).

A future research question, which we did not explore, should be how such programs must evolve in the context of a significantly changed health care and funding environment. Changes in Ryan White funding and the Afford-able Care Act will provide tremendous opportunities to serve PLWH better but will also require adjustment by organizations serving PLWH. Also, we did not explore the challenges associated with reaching particular groups that are most often not engaged in ongoing HIV care in the United States (e.g., youth), and future studies could examine the suitability of approaches for reaching such groups (Hall, Frazier, et al. 2013; Maulsby et al. 2015).

Linkage to and retention in ongoing primary HIV care is a prerequisite for healthy, stable lives for PLWH and for achieving the suppressed viral loads that prevent further HIV transmission (Cohen et al. 2011). To stem the domestic HIV epidemic, a wide range of biomedical (e.g., HAART, PrEP, treatment of STIs), behavioral (e.g., medication adherence), and structural (e.g., housing) interventions are necessary. Since the start of Positive Charge, more groups have joined the effort to link individuals to care and retain them in care (Mugavero et al. 2013). Our sincere hope is that these findings can be used to inform program design and provide some insights as every program's inevi-table course corrections arise. Specifically, we hope that the work described in this book is informative about key program inputs necessary for success, re-alistic depictions of challenges, and candidly presented lessons learned. As the work of linkage to and retention in care in the United States is just begin-ning, future studies examining this process will greatly add to nascent cur-rent knowledge and build on the insights presented here.

Appendixes

The following appendixes are the semistructured case study interview guide (appendix A) and the online network collaboration survey (appendix B). These are the instruments used to gather data for these case studies. They are included here as a reference not only to inform the reader but also for other implementation researchers potentially interested in exploring similar research questions.

As described in the methods, the semistructured interview guide was developed by the Johns Hopkins University research team and adapted slightly based on each individual site project. The flow and content of the questions were updated iteratively as more interviews were completed and saturation around particular themes occurred or respondents' insights brought new queries to light. The survey questions were adapted from similar studies on HIV and interorganizational collaboration in New York City and Baltimore (Messeri and Kiperman 1994; Kwait et al. 2001). Although reliability and validity testing was not conducted, the survey questions have strong face validity and were reviewed by network analysis experts. Additionally, asking respondents about a "checklist" of possible organizations they have worked with is a widely used method for collecting network data. These questions are included as appendix B.

Appendix A
Semistructured Case Study Interview Guide

1. Describe your organization and the type of services you provide to PLWH (ice breaker).
2. Please tell me about [your organization].
3. How is your organization involved with [your project]?

Work with clients:

4. How does your organization identify PLWH who are out of care? *Probe on strategies (e.g., peer navigators or CHWs).*
5. Could you take me through how your project links out-of-care individuals to care? *Probe on strategies.*
6. Once an individual is linked to care, how does your organization ensure these individuals stay in care? *Probe on strategies (e.g., motivational interviewing).*
7. How did your organization determine ways of finding, linking, and retaining individuals in care?
8. *(If peer navigators were mentioned)* From your work, can you tell me what makes a successful peer/health navigator?

Within organization:

9. What has changed since [your project] began at your organization?
10. Are there changes that you wish had been implemented, but were not? Can you tell me about those? *(If changes mentioned, probe: how would such a change have helped you?)*
11. How did your organization identify out-of-care clients before [your project]? *Probe for changes.*
12. How did your organization link clients into care before [your project]? *Probe for changes.*
13. How did your organization retain clients into care before [your project]? *Probe for changes.*
14. Overall, is [your project] going as it was planned? How so? [If no] Why not? *Probe for changes and reasons why.*

Partner organizations:

15. What outside organizations or agencies do you work with most for [your project]?
16. What does each organization do for [the project]?
17. Could you tell me about your experience working with each organization? *Probe for formal contracts vs. informal connections; sharing of client information.*

Project facilitators and barriers:
18. What have been your biggest barriers to doing this work? *Probe for program or strategy-specific barriers.*
19. What successful strategies has [your organization] used to overcome these barriers?
20. Can you describe any unsuccessful strategies [your organization] tried?
21. Could you describe factors that have helped [your organization] in doing this work?
22. *(If applicable)* As your program works with [specific hard-to-reach population], what has [your organization]'s experience been in reaching these individuals?

Project context:
23. In your opinion, how has [your project] affected your organization? *Probe: Internal structural changes.*
24. Have there been any unexpected or unintended outcomes of [your project]?
25. Could you tell us about services you would like to offer or refer PLWH to that are not easily available, if any?
26. Could you tell us about anything you'd like to have that could help you do your job better?
27. How do you feel that specific policies in your organization have affected your work? *If respondent is knowledgeable about policy, probe on provider, local, and national policies.*
28. If you could change three policies to enhance your work, what changes would you make?

Recent legislation:
29. How do you foresee the new health care law affecting your work? *Probe on services offered.*
30. Do you see new LGBT-friendly policies affecting your work? *Probe: If yes, please describe how.*

Closing:
31. Is there anything else you would like to share with me about your experiences with [your project]?

Appendix B
Network Collaboration Survey Questions

The following questions were included in online surveys sent to "admin" respondents:

Organizational characteristics
What is the legal/fiscal designation of [your organization] (choose one)?
- Public
- Private not for profit
- Private for profit
- Other (specify)

Which category best describes [your organization] (choose one)?
- Hospital-based clinic
- Federal or state qualified community health center
- Federal or state qualified community mental health center
- Local/County/City/State Health Department
- Home health hospice agency
- Other health service agency (Specify)
- Local/County/State Social Services Department
- Other social services organization (Specify)
- Other (Specify)

What is the estimated total annual operating budget for [your organization]?
What is the estimated annual total operating budget for [your organization]'s HIV specific services?
How many PLWH were served by [your organization]? If you are not sure of the exact number of PLWH served, please provide a "best guess" estimate.
Briefly describe the client community served by [your organization]
How many paid employees did [your organization] have in [most recent fiscal year]?
How many volunteers did [your organization] have in [most recent fiscal year]?

The following questions were asked of all respondents through an online survey:

Introduction
Name of organization you work for
Organization address
Your initials
Your job title
Your phone extension
Length of time you worked for this organization

Description of Services

Which of the following services does [your organization] provide for PLWH? Please select all that apply.

- STI/HIV counseling and testing
- HIV primary care
- HIV case management
- HIV outreach and linkage to care services
- HIV peer support/peer mentoring services
- Other health services (e.g., non-HIV primary care, dental services, mental health services provided by a licensed professional (individual or group services, not including general counseling by non-professionals or support groups)). Please specify below:
- Counseling services (e.g., general counseling provided by non-professionals, HIV adherence counseling, nutrition counseling). Please specify below:
- Education (e.g., HIV self-management). Please specify below:
- HIV prevention services. Please specify below:
- Assistance with providing entitlement services
- Substance abuse treatment
- Housing services
- Other support services, such as daycare for children, transportation services, food distribution, and legal services. Please specify below:
- Smoking cessation services
- Training. Please specify below:
- Other (specify):
- None

Which of these activities have been added or augmented as a result of [program name]? Please select all that apply.

- STI/HIV counseling and testing
- HIV primary care
- HIV case management
- HIV outreach and linkage to care services
- HIV peer support/peer mentoring services
- Other health services (e.g., non-HIV primary care, dental services, mental health services provided by a licensed professional (individual or group services, not including general counseling by non-professionals or support groups)). Please specify below:
- Counseling services (e.g., general counseling provided by non-professionals, HIV adherence counseling, nutrition counseling). Please specify below:
- Education (e.g., HIV self-management). Please specify below:
- HIV prevention services. Please specify below:
- Assistance with providing entitlement services
- Substance abuse treatment
- Housing services
- Other support services, such as daycare for children, transportation services, food distribution, and legal services. Please specify below:
- Smoking cessation services
- Training. Please specify below:
- Other (specify):
- None

Collaboration (yes/no) with other organizations in the local PC network

This section was repeated for each member of the local PC network.

Did your organization collaborate with [partner organization] in the implementation of [project name]?
- Yes
- No

If yes, then the following questions were asked about the partner organization:

How often did your organization engage in the following linkages with [partner organization] as part of [project name]?
- Refer participants to this agency
- Receive participants referred from this agency to your organization
- Discuss services offered by this agency with participants
- Assist participants with accessing services offered by this agency
- Receive participants who got assistance from this agency in accessing services at your organization
- Attend regularly scheduled meetings
- Participate in joint conference calls
- Exchange information with staff of the agency (such as phone calls or email)
- Provide consultation or technical assistance to the agency
- Receive consultation or technical assistance from the agency
- Share resources such as supplies or transportation. Please specify:
- Other (specify)

Did [your organization] engage in any of the following linkages with [partner organization] as part of [project name]?
- Some of our staff is located at their agency
- Some of their staff is located at our facility
- Have a formal contract agreement or MoU with the agency
- Other (specify)
- None of the above

When [project name] participants were receiving services from both [your organization] and [partner organization], how often was HIV care-related information about the client exchanged?
- Not relevant for this collaboration
- Not applicable because of HIPAA or legal constraints
- Never (allowable but never occurs)
- Rarely
- Sometimes
- Very often
- Always

In the six months before [project name], how often did your organization engage in the following linkages with [partner organization]? Please do not include collaboration that may have occurred in preparation for [project name].
- Refer clients to this agency
- Receive participants referred from this agency to your organization
- Discuss services offered by this agency with participants

- Assist participants with accessing services offered by this agency
- Receive participants who got assistance from this agency in accessing services at your organization
- Attend regularly scheduled meetings
- Participate in joint conference calls
- Exchange information with staff of the agency (such as phone calls or email)
- Provide consultation or technical assistance to the agency
- Receive consultation or technical assistance from the agency
- Share resources such as supplies or transportation. Please specify:
- Other (specify)

In the six months before [project name], did [your organization] engage in any of the following linkages with [partner organization]? Please select all that apply. Please do not include collaboration that may have occurred in preparation for [project name].

- Some of our staff is located at their agency
- Some of their staff is located at our facility
- Have a formal contract agreement or MoU with the agency
- Other (specify)
- None of the above

Additional agencies

Were you working with other organizations to implement [project name]?

- Yes
- No

Please name these organizations and describe how you were working with them to implement [project name].

6 months all organizations

In the six months before [project name], did your organization work with any of the following organizations to link PLWH into HIV care and treatment? Please select all that apply. You may select more than one answer. If you work for the organization, please do not select it. Please do not include collaboration that might have occurred in preparation for [project name].

- Partner organization 1
- Partner organization 2
- Partner organization 3 (etc.)
- Other (specify)
- None of the above

References

Althoff, K. N., et al. (2012). "US trends in antiretroviral therapy use, HIV RNA plasma viral loads, and CD4 T-lymphocyte cell counts among HIV-infected persons, 2000 to 2008." *Annals of Internal Medicine* 157(5): 325–335.

amfAR (2013). Syringe Exchange Program Coverage in the United States—July 2013. www .amfar.org/uploadedFiles/_amfarorg/Articles/In_The_Community/2013/July%202013%20 SEP%20Map%20.pdf.

Andersen, M., et al. (2007). "Retaining women in HIV medical care." *Journal of the Association of Nurses in AIDS Care* 18(3): 33–41.

Antiretroviral Therapy Cohort Collaboration (2008). "Life expectancy of individuals on combination antiretroviral therapy in high-income countries: a collaborative analysis of 14 cohort studies." *Lancet* 372(9635): 293–299.

ATLAS.ti (2013). Software. Berlin, Germany, GmbH.

Bhaskaran, K., et al. (2008). "Changes in the risk of death after HIV seroconversion compared with mortality in the general population." *JAMA* 300(1): 51–59.

Borgatti, S. P., et al. (2002). Ucinet for Windows: Software for Social Network Analysis. Harvard, Cambridge, MA, Analytic Technologies.

Bradford, J. B. (2007). "The promise of outreach for engaging and retaining out-of-care persons in HIV medical care." *AIDS Patient Care and STDs* 21(S1): S85-91.

California Department of Public Health (CDPH) (2013). HIV/AIDS Surveillance in California: December 2013 Semi Annual Report. www.cdph.ca.gov/programs/aids/Documents/Dec_2013 _Semi_Annual%20Report.pdf.

Cambiano, V., et al. (2014). "Predicted levels of HIV drug resistance: potential impact of expanding diagnosis, retention, and eligibility criteria for antiretroviral therapy initiation." *AIDS* 28: S15-23.

CASCADE Collaboration (2003). "Determinants of survival following HIV-1 seroconversion after the introduction of HAART." *Lancet* 362(9392): 1267–1274.

Centerforce (2011). Form 990. Return of Organization Exempt from Income Tax. https://bulk .resource.org/irs.gov/eo/2012_01_EO/51-0209800_990_201106.pdf.

Centers for Disease Control and Prevention (2011a). HIV Surveillance Report: Diagnoses of HIV Infection and AIDS in the United States and Dependent Areas, vol. 23. www.cdc.gov /hiv/library/reports/surveillance/2011/surveillance_Report_vol_23.html.

Centers for Disease Control and Prevention (2011b). "Vital signs: HIV prevention through care and treatment—United States." *MMWR Morbidity and Mortality Weekly Report* 60(47): 1618.

Centers for Disease Control and Prevention (2012a). HIV Surveillance Report: Diagnoses of HIV Infection in the United States and Dependent Areas, vol. 24. www.cdc.gov/hiv/library /reports/surveillance.

Centers for Disease Control and Prevention (2012b). HIV Surveillance Supplemental Report: Monitoring Selected National HIV Prevention and Care Objectives by Using HIV Surveillance Data—United States and 6 Dependent Areas—2011, vol. 18. www.cdc.gov/hiv/pdf/2011 _Monitoring_HIV_Indicators_HSSR_FINAL.pdf.

Centers for Disease Control and Prevention (2013). CDC Fact Sheet: HIV in the United States: The Stages of Care. www.cdc.gov/nchhstp/newsroom/docs/HIV-Stages-of-Care-Factsheet -508.pdf.

Cohen, M. S., et al. (2011). "Prevention of HIV-1 infection with early antiretroviral therapy." *New England Journal of Medicine* 365(6): 493–505.

Coleman, S. M., et al. (2009). "Sexual risk behavior and behavior change among persons newly diagnosed with HIV: the impact of targeted outreach interventions among hard-to-reach populations." *AIDS Patient Care and STDs* 23(8): 639–645.

Conviser, R., and Pounds, M. (2002). "The role of ancillary services in client-centred systems of care." *AIDS Care* 14(S1): 119–131.

Craw, J. A., et al. (2008). "Brief strengths-based case management promotes entry into HIV medical care: results of the Antiretroviral Treatment Access Study-II." *JAIDS Journal of Acquired Immune Deficiency Syndromes* 47(5): 597–606.

Das, M., et al. (2010). "Decreases in community viral load are accompanied by reductions in new HIV infections in San Francisco." *PLoS One* 5(6): e11068.

Department of Health and Hospitals State of Louisiana (2015). Louisiana Medicaid Enrollment Trends Reports. www.dhh.state.la.us/index.cfm/page/1275.

Detels, R., et al. (1998). "Effectiveness of potent antiretroviral therapy on time to AIDS and death in men with known HIV infection duration." *JAMA* 280(17): 1497–1503.

Deutskens, E., et al. (2006). "An assessment of equivalence between online and mail surveys in service research." *Journal of Service Research* 8(4): 346–355.

Dryfoos, J. G. (1994). *Full-Service Schools: A Revolution in Health and Social Services for Children, Youth, and Families.* San Francisco, Jossey-Bass.

Eysenbach, G., and Wyatt, J. (2002). "Using the Internet for surveys and health research." *Journal of Medical Internet Research* 4(2): e13.

Foust, E., and Clymore, J. (2011). Epidemiologic Profile for HIV/STD Prevention & Care Planning. Raleigh, NC, Division of Public Health, NC Department of Health & Human Services. http://epi.publichealth.nc.gov/cd/stds/figures/Epi_Profile_2011.pdf.

Gardner, E. M., et al. (2011). "The spectrum of engagement in HIV care and its relevance to test-and-treat strategies for prevention of HIV infection." *Clinical Infectious Diseases* 52(6): 793–800.

Gardner, L. I., et al. (2005). "Efficacy of a brief case management intervention to link recently diagnosed HIV-infected persons to care." *AIDS* 19(4): 423–431.

Gupta, R. K., et al. (2012). "Global trends in antiretroviral resistance in treatment-naive individuals with HIV after rollout of antiretroviral treatment in resource-limited settings: a global collaborative study and meta-regression analysis." *Lancet* 380(9849): 1250–1258.

Haley, D. F., et al. (2014). "Retention strategies and factors associated with missed visits among low income women at increased risk of HIV acquisition in the US (HPTN 064)." *AIDS Patient Care and STDs* 28(4): 206–217.

Hall, H. I., et al. (2012). "Retention in care of adults and adolescents living with HIV in 13 US areas." *JAIDS Journal of Acquired Immune Deficiency Syndromes* 60(1): 77–82.

Hall, H. I., Frazier, E. L., et al. (2013). "Differences in human immunodeficiency virus care and treatment among subpopulations in the United States." *JAMA Internal Medicine* 173(14): 1337–1344.

Hall, H. I., Tang, T., et al. (2013). "HIV care visits and time to viral suppression, 19 U.S. jurisdictions, and implications for treatment, prevention and the National HIV/AIDS Strategy." *PLoS One* 8(12): e84318.

HBHC (2010). Form 990. Return of Organization Exempt from Income Tax: Public Disclosure Copy. www.howardbrown.org/uploadedFiles/About_Us/2010%20Form%20990%20HBHC .pdf.

Herwehe, J., et al. (2011). "Implementation of an innovative, integrated electronic medical record (EMR) and public health information exchange for HIV/AIDS." *Journal of the American Medical Informatics Association*, amiajnl-2011-000412.

Hightow-Weidman, L. B., Jones, K., et al. (2011). "Early linkage and retention in care: findings from the outreach, linkage, and retention in care initiative among young men of color who have sex with men." *AIDS Patient Care and STDs* 25(S1): S31-38.

Hightow-Weidman, L. B., Smith, J. C., et al. (2011). "Keeping them in 'STYLE': finding, linking, and retaining young HIV-positive black and Latino men who have sex with men in care." *AIDS Patient Care and STDs* 25(1): 37–45.

Hsieh, H.-F., and Shannon, S. E. (2005). "Three approaches to qualitative content analysis." *Qualitative Health Research* 15(9): 1277–1288.

Illinois Department of Health (2013). Illinois HIV/AIDS/STD Monthly Surveillance Update. Springfield, IL. www.idph.state.il.us/aids/Surv_Report_0613.pdf.

Jones, N., et al. (2004). "Collaborating for mental health services in Wales: a process evaluation." *Public Administration* 82(1): 109–121.

Kaiser Family Foundation (2012). Total Federal Grant Funding. http://kff.org/hivaids/state -indicator/total-federal-grant-funding.

Kempf, M.-C., et al. (2010). "A qualitative study of the barriers and facilitators to retention-in-care among HIV-positive women in the rural southeastern United States: implications for targeted interventions." *AIDS Patient Care and STDs* 24(8): 515–520.

Kim, J. J., et al. (2014). "The national evaluation of a multisite access to care initiative: AIDS United's access to care initiative." *AIDS Education and Prevention* 26: 429–444.

Krantz, J. H., et al. (1997). "Comparing the results of laboratory and World-Wide Web samples on the determinants of female attractiveness." *Behavior Research Methods, Instruments, & Computers* 29(2): 264–269.

Kwait, J., et al. (2001). "Interorganizational relationships among HIV/AIDS service organizations in Baltimore: a network analysis." *Journal of Urban Health Bulletin of the New York Academy of Medicine* 78(3): 468–487.

Lincoln, Y. S., and Guba, E. G. (1985). *Naturalistic Inquiry*. Newbury Park, CA, SAGE.

Lippitt, R., and Van Til, J. (1981). "Can we achieve a collaborative community? Issues, imperatives, potentials." *Journal of Voluntary Action Research* 10(3/4): 7–17.

Louisiana Office of Public Health (2011). Louisiana Department of Health and Hospitals Office of Public Health STD/HIV Program Report. http://new.dhh.louisiana.gov.

LSU (2009). The LSU Hospitals and Clinics. www.lsuhospitals.org/docs/LSU_AnnualReport2011 .pdf.

LSU Health (2015). Earl King Long Medical Center Is Now Closed. www.lsuhospitals.org/EKL .aspx.

Mallinson, R. K., et al. (2007). "The provider role in client engagement in HIV care." *AIDS Patient Care and STDs* 21(S1): S77-84.

Manning, K. (1997). "Authenticity in constructivist inquiry: methodological considerations without prescription." *Qualitative Inquiry* 3(1): 93–115.

Mattessich, P. W., and Monsey, B. R. (1992). *Collaboration: What Makes It Work. A Review of Research Literature on Factors Influencing Successful Collaboration.* St. Paul, Minnesota, Wilder Research.

Maulsby, C., et al. (2015). "Positive Charge: filling the gaps in the US HIV continuum of care." *AIDS and Behavior*, Feb. 12 [Epub ahead of print].

Messeri, P., et al. (1994). Seven Cities HIV Early Intervention Demonstration Projects: Second Year Update: Chicago, New York City and Washington, D.C. Report prepared under a Co-operative Agreement with the Centers for Disease Control and Prevention.

Metsch, L. R., et al. (2008). "HIV transmission risk behaviors among HIV-infected persons who are successfully linked to care." *Clinical Infectious Diseases* 47(4): 577–584.

MNHC (2009). Form 990. Return of Organization Exempt from Income Tax. https://bulk.resource.org/irs.gov/eo/2010_12_EO/94-2284365_990_200912.pdf.

Moore, R. D., and Bartlett, J. G. (2011). "Dramatic decline in the HIV-1 RNA level over calendar time in a large urban HIV practice." *Clinical Infectious Diseases* 53(6): 600–604.

Mugavero, M. J., et al. (2013). "The state of engagement in HIV care in the United States: from cascade to continuum to control." *Clinical Infectious Diseases* 57(8): 1164–1171.

Myers, J. E., et al. (2012). "Transmitted drug resistance among antiretroviral-naive patients with established HIV type 1 infection in Santo Domingo, Dominican Republic and review of the Latin American and Caribbean literature." *AIDS Research and Human Retroviruses* 28(7): 667–674.

Naar-King, S., et al. (2007). "Retention in care of persons newly diagnosed with HIV: outcomes of the Outreach Initiative." *AIDS Patient Care and STDs* 21(S1): S40-48.

NASTAD (2012). National ADAP Monitoring Project Annual Report. www.nastad.org/Docs/021503_National%20ADAP%20Monitoring%20Project%20Annual%20Report%20-%20August%202012.pdf.

NASTAD (2014). National ADAP Monitoring Project: Annual Report. www.nastad.org/docs/NASTAD%20National%20ADAP%20Monitoring%20Project%20Annual%20Report%20-%20February%202014.pdf.

Nathanson, A. T., and Reinert, S. E. (1999). "Windsurfing injuries: results of a paper- and Internet-based survey." *Wilderness & Environmental Medicine* 10(4): 218–225.

New York City Department of Health and Mental Hygiene (2012). HIV Surveillance Annual Report, 2012. www.nyc.gov/html/doh/downloads/pdf/dires/surveillance-report-dec-2013.pdf.

Olatosi, B. A., et al. (2009). "Patterns of engagement in care by HIV-infected adults: South Carolina, 2004–2006." *AIDS* 23(6): 725–730.

ONAP (2010). National HIV/AIDS Strategy for the United States. Washington, DC, The White House. www.whitehouse.gov/sites/default/files/uploads/NHAS.pdf.

Palella, F. J., et al. (1998). "Declining morbidity and mortality among patients with advanced human immunodeficiency virus infection." *New England Journal of Medicine* 338: 853–860.

Parmigiani, A., and Rivera-Santos, M. (2011). "Clearing a path through the forest: a meta-review of interorganizational relationships." *Journal of Management* 37(4): 1108–1136.

Perkins, D., et al. (2008). "Assessing HIV care and unmet need: eight data bases and a bit of perseverance." *AIDS Care* 20(3): 318–326.

Provan, K. G., et al. (2003). "Building community capacity around chronic disease services through a collaborative interorganizational network." *Health Education & Behavior* 30(6): 646–662.

Rajabiun, S., et al. (2007). "Program design and evaluation strategies for the Special Projects of National Significance Outreach Initiative." *AIDS Patient Care and STDs* 21(S1): S9-19.

Rebeiro, P., et al. (2013). "Retention among North American HIV-infected persons in clinical care, 2000–2008." *JAIDS Journal of Acquired Immune Deficiency Syndromes* 62(3): 356–362.

San Francisco Department of Public Health (SFDPF) (2012). HIV/AIDS Epidemiology Annual Report. www.sfdph.org/dph/files/reports/RptsHIVAIDS/AnnualReport2012.pdf.

Schmidt, W. C. (1997). "World-Wide Web survey research: benefits, potential problems, and solutions." *Behavior Research Methods, Instruments, & Computers* 29(2): 274–279.

SFAF (2010). Form 990. Return of Organization Exempt from Income Tax. www.sfaf.org/about-us /financial-information/tax-return-form-990-year2010-2011-sanfranciscoaidsfoundation.pdf.

Sprague, C., and Simon, S. E. (2014). "Understanding HIV care delays in the US South and the role of the social-level in HIV care engagement/retention: a qualitative study." *International Journal for Equity in Health* 2: 3.

Thomas, J. C., et al. (2007). "An interagency network perspective on HIV prevention." *Sexually Transmitted Diseases* 34(2): 71–75.

Thompson, M. A., et al. (2012). "Guidelines for improving entry into and retention in care and antiretroviral adherence for persons with HIV: evidence-based recommendations from an International Association of Physicians in AIDS Care panel." *Annals of Internal Medicine* 156(11): 817–833.

Torian, L., et al. (2011). "HIV surveillance—United States, 1981–2008." *MMWR Morbidity and Mortality Weekly Report* 60: 689–693. www.cdc.gov/mmwr/preview/mmwrhtml/mm6021a2.htm.

Ulett, K. B., et al. (2009). "The therapeutic implications of timely linkage and early retention in HIV care." *AIDS Patient Care and STDs* 23(1): 41–49.

U.S. Census Bureau (2010a). State & County QuickFacts. http://quickfacts.census.gov/qfd/ states/17/1714000.html.

U.S. Census Bureau (2010b). State & County QuickFacts. http://quickfacts.census.gov/qfd/ states/36/3651000.html.

U.S. Census Bureau (2015). State Totals: Vintage 2014. www.census.gov/popest/data/state/totals /2014/index.html.

Wohl, A. R., Galvan, F. H., et al. (2011). "Do social support, stress, disclosure and stigma influence retention in HIV care for Latino and African American men who have sex with men and women?" *AIDS and Behavior* 15(6): 1098–1110.

Wohl, A. R., Garland, W. H., et al. (2011). "A youth-focused case management intervention to engage and retain young gay men of color in HIV care." *AIDS Care* 23(8): 988–997.

World Health Organization (2014). World Health Statistics 2014: Part III—Global Health Indicators. www.who.int/gho/publications/world_health_statistics/EN_WHS2014_Part3.pdf.

Wright, E. R., and Shuff, I. M. (1995). "Specifying the integration of mental health and primary health care services for persons with HIV/AIDS: the Indiana integration of care project." *Social Networks* 17(3): 319–340.

Yin, R. K. (2009). *Case Study Research*. Thousand Oaks, CA, SAGE.

Index

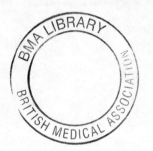